Melvin Delgado, PhD
Editor

Latino Elders and the Twenty-First Century: Issues and Challenges for Culturally Competent Research and Practice

Latino Elders and the Twenty-First Century: Issues and Challenges for Culturally Competent Research and Practice has been co-published simultaneously as *Journal of Gerontological Social Work*, Volume 30, Numbers 1/2 1998.

Pre-publication
REVIEWS,
COMMENTARIES,
EVALUATIONS . . .

"**A**s we enter the new millennium, *Latino Elders in the Twenty-First Century: Issues and Challenges for Culturally Competent Research and Practice* makes an invaluable contribution towards enhancing Social Work's understanding of sociocultural issues relevant to addressing the social needs of Latino elders. Social Workers will find a rich array of articles that identify current research issues and practice principles that will guide their work with Latino elders across ethnic specific groups.

This special issue makes a significant contribution to the field of gerontological social work by providing a culturally competent research and practice framework for understanding the health and human service needs of the Latino elder population. The reader interested in the social work needs of Latino elders is provided with a sound, thoughtful analysis of the current social policy and clinical practice issues necessary for the development of culturally competent services."

Edgar Colon, DSW
Associate Professor of Social Work
Southern Connecticut State University
New Haven, CT

"**E**very social worker will need to read this special issue focusing on the challenges Latino elders present for culturally competent gerontological social work in the 21st Century. This special edition edited by Dr. Melvin Delgado is a long overdue examination of a neglected and misunderstood population, Latino elders. As the fastest growing older population in the United States, it is appalling that we lack even the most basic demographic data on this population. This makes this special issue an even more important contribution to ethnogerontological social work practice.

Throughout this excellent series of articles, one major theme is reiterated, namely, the lack of culturally sensitive research and scholarship on Latino elders. This collection goes a long way towards filling this gap. Several articles report on unique research related to Latino service utilization, caregiving patterns, and natural support networks. The volume also poses many significant questions for further research and scholarship on Latino elders, and if it is successful in stimulating inquiry into these issues, we may see another publication on Latino elders in the not too distant future.

There is a good progression in the articles from broad cultural issues to specific problems that social workers will have to address if they plan to meet the needs of this diverse population. In the introductory article, Applewhite points out the increasing needs of Latino elders given the significant erosion of the Latino community's formal and informal safety net. He states, ". . . the presumed automatic guarantees of emotional, economic and social support for elderly Latinos traditionally provided by the extended family have slowly eroded over time due to such factors as mobility, acculturation, prohibitive costs, and the multiple stresses on elderly caregivers." This presents significant issues of concerns for social workers who are expected to serve a diverse, bicultural and sometimes bilingual, impoverished, and somewhat isolated population of Latino elders who may be reluctant to utilize culturally insensitive and unresponsive health, mental health, and social services.

Applewhite echoes another important theme present throughout the articles, namely that theories of aging do not accurately reflect the Latino elders cultural or ethnic experiences. Culturally competent social workers need to develop ethnogerontological knowledge, values and skills that more accurately and sensitively reflect the needs of Latino elders. Mizio's article on culturally sensitive staff development programs lays out an excellent conceptual framework for a training curriculum that, if implemented, could lead to skilled culturally competent social workers.

Paulino examines a fast growing Latino population, the Dominican immigrant community. She describes the special needs of Dominican elders by reporting on a focused group that brought out significant cultural factors in the lives of Dominican elders such as the importance of a Dominican identity, the "returning home" theme, "circular" migration patterns, religious beliefs, and family caregiving patterns, all issues that impact on service delivery to this population.

I especially enjoyed Sanchez-Ayendez's well-conceptualized qualitative study on middle-aged Puerto Rican women as caregivers. It was a thoughtful and insightful study that captured the Latina "sandwich" generation with all its cultural imperatives and stressors. The two articles comparing white, African-American and Puerto Rican caregivers are important cross-cultural comparison studies which highlight the subtle differences and commonalities between these groups. Since most of the literature on substance abuse examines the problem primarily from the adult Latino males point of view, Kail and De La Rosa's examination of the impact of alcohol and other drugs on Latino elders is unique and useful for practitioners. Again what makes this issue so valuable are the articles reporting on exciting new research that informs gerontological social work practice in a very special, practitioner-friendly way.

In general, I give this special issue my blessing and look forward to its publication and utilization in my courses such as Human Behavior in the Social Environment and Multicultural Social Work Practice.

I appreciate the opportunity to review this work, and congratulate the *Journal*, its editors, and contributors on making such an important contribution to improving the quality of life for all Latinos."

Carmen Ortiz Hendricks, DSW
Hunter College School of Social Work
New York, NY

Latino Elders
and the Twenty-First Century:
Issues and Challenges
for Culturally Competent
Research and Practice

Latino Elders and the Twenty-First Century: Issues and Challenges for Culturally Competent Research and Practice has been co-published simultaneously as *Journal of Gerontological Social Work*, Volume 30, Numbers 1/2 1998.

The *Journal of Gerontological Social Work* Monographic "Separates"

Below is a list of "separates," which in serials librarianship means a special issue simultaneously published as a special journal issue or double-issue *and* as a "separate" hardbound monograph. (This is a format which we also call a "Docuserial.")

"Separates" are published because specialized libraries or professionals may wish to purchase a specific thematic issue by itself in a format which can be separately cataloged and shelved, as opposed to purchasing the journal on an on-going basis. Faculty members may also more easily consider a "separate" for classroom adoption.

"Separates" are carefully classified separately with the major book jobbers so that the journal tie-in can be noted on new book order slips to avoid duplicate purchasing.

You may wish to visit Haworth's website at . . .

http://www.haworthpressinc.com

. . . to search our online catalog for complete tables of contents of these separates and related publications.

You may also call 1-800-HAWORTH (outside US/Canada: 607-722-5857), or Fax 1-800-895-0582 (outside US/Canada: 607-771-0012), or e-mail at:

getinfo@haworthpressinc.com

Latino Elders and the Twenty-First Century: Issues and Challenges for Culturally Competent Research and Practice, edited by Melvin Delgado (JGSW 30(1/2), Available Fall 1998) *"Explores the challenges that gerontological social work will encounter as it attempts to meet the needs of the growing number of Latino elders utilizing culturally competent principles."*

Dignity and Old Age, edited by Robert Disch, Rose Dobrof and Harry R. Moody (JGSW 29(2/3), 1998) *"Challenges us to uphold the right to age with dignity, which is embedded in the heart and soul of every man and woman."* (H. James Towey, President, Commission on Aging with Dignity, Tallahassee, FL)

Intergenerational Approaches in Aging: Implications for Education, Policy and Practice, edited by Kevin Brabazon and Robert Disch (JGSW 28(1/2/3), 1997) *"Provides a wealth of concrete examples of areas in which intergenerational perspectives and knowledge are needed."* (Robert C. Atchley, PhD, Director, Scribbs Gerontology Center, Miami University)

Social Work Response to the White House Conference on Aging: From Issues to Actions, edited by Constance Corley Saltz (JGSW 27(3), 1997) *"Provides a framework for the discussion of issues relevant to social work values and practice, including productive aging, quality of life, the psychological needs of older persons, and family issues."* (Jordan I. Kosberg, PhD, Professor and PhD Program Coordinator, School of Social Work, Florida International University, North Miami, FL)

Special Aging Populations and Systems Linkages, edited by M. Joanna Mellor (JGSW 25(1/2), 1996) *"An invaluable tool for anyone working with older persons with special needs."* (Irene Gutheil, DSW, Associate Professor, Graduate School of Social Service, Fordham University)

New Developments in Home Care Services for the Elderly: Innovations in Policy, Program, and Practice, edited by Lenard W. Kaye (JGSW 24(3/4), 1995) *"An excellent compilation. . . . Especially pertinent to the functions of administrators, supervisors, and case managers in home care. . . . Highly recommended for every home care agency and a must for administrators and middle managers."* (Geriatric Nursing Book Review)

Geriatric Social Work Education, edited by M. Joanna Mellor and Renee Solomon (JGSW 18(3/4), 1992) *"Serves as a foundation upon which educators and fieldwork instructors can build courses that incorporate more aging content."* (SciTech Book News)

Vision and Aging: Issues in Social Work Practice, edited by Nancy D. Weber (JGSW 17(3/4), 1992) *"For those involved in vision rehabilitation programs, the book provides practical information and should stimulate readers to revise their present programs of care." (Journal of Vision Rehabilitation)*

Health Care of the Aged: Needs, Policies, and Services, edited by Abraham Monk (JGSW 15(3/4), 1990) *"The chapters reflect firsthand experience and are competent and informative. Readers . . . will find the book rewarding and useful. The text is timely, appropriate, and well-presented." (Health & Social Work)*

Twenty-Five Years of the Life Review: Theoretical and Practical Considerations, edited by Robert Disch (JGSW 12(3/4), 1989) *This practical and thought-provoking book examines the history and concept of the life review.*

Gerontological Social Work: International Perspectives, edited by Merl C. Hokenstad, Jr. and Katherine A. Kendall (JGSW 12(1/2), 1988) *"Makes a very useful contribution in examining the changing role of the social work profession in serving the elderly." (Journal of the International Federation on Ageing)*

Gerontological Social Work Practice with Families: A Guide to Practice Issues and Service Delivery, edited by Rose Dobrof (JGSW 10(1/2), 1987) *An in-depth examination of the importance of family relationships within the context of social work practice with the elderly.*

Ethnicity and Gerontological Social Work, edited by Rose Dobrof (JGSW 9(4), 1987) *"Addresses the issues of ethnicity with great sensitivity. Most of the topics addressed here are rarely addressed in other literature." (Dr. Milada Disman, Department of Behavioral Science, University of Toronto)*

Social Work and Alzheimer's Disease, edited by Rose Dobrof (JGSW 9(2), 1986) *"New and innovative social work roles with Alzheimer's victims and their families in both hospital and non-hospital settings." (Continuing Education Update)*

Gerontological Social Work Practice in the Community, edited by George S. Getzel and M. Joanna Mellor (JGSW 8(3/4), 1985) *"A wealth of information for all practitioners who deal with the elderly. An excellent reference for faculty, administrators, clinicians, and graduate students in nursing and other service professions who work with the elderly." (American Journal of Care for the Aging)*

Gerontological Social Work in Home Health Care, edited by Rose Dobrof (JGSW 7(4), 1984) *"A useful window onto the home health care scene in terms of current forms of service provided to the elderly and the direction of social work practice in this field today." (PRIDE Institute Journal)*

The Uses of Reminiscence: New Ways of Working with Older Adults, edited by Marc Kaminsky (JGSW 7(1/2), 1984) *"Rich in ideas for anyone working with life review groups." (Guidepost)*

A Healthy Old Age: A Sourcebook for Health Promotion with Older Adults, edited by Stephanie FallCreek and Molly K. Mettler (JGSW 6(2/3), 1984) *"An outstanding text on the 'how-tos' of health promotion for elderly persons." (Physical Therapy)*

Gerontological Social Work Practice in Long-Term Care, edited by George S. Getzel and M. Joanna Mellor (JGSW 5(1/2), 1983) *"Veteran practitioners and graduate social work students will find the book insightful and a valuable prescriptive guide to the dos and don'ts of practice in their daily work." (The Gerontologist)*

Latino Elders and the Twenty-First Century: Issues and Challenges for Culturally Competent Research and Practice

Melvin Delgado, PhD
Editor

Latino Elders and the Twenty-First Century: Issues and Challenges for Culturally Competent Research and Practice has been co-published simultaneously as *Journal of Gerontological Social Work*, Volume 30, Numbers 1/2 1998.

The Haworth Press, Inc.
New York • London

Latino Elders and the Twenty-First Century: Issues and Challenges for Culturally Competent Research and Practice has been co-published simultaneously as *Journal of Gerontological Social Work*™, Volume 30, Numbers 1/2 1998.

The development, preparation, and publication of this work has been undertaken with great care. However, the publisher, employees, editors, and agents of The Haworth Press and all imprints of The Haworth Press, Inc., including The Haworth Medical Press® and Pharmaceutical Products Press®, are not responsible for any errors contained herein or for consequences that may ensue from use of materials or information contained in this work. Opinions expressed by the author(s) are not necessarily those of The Haworth Press, Inc.

The Haworth Press, Inc., 10 Alice Street, Binghamton, NY 13904-1580 USA

Cover design by Thomas J. Mayshock Jr.

Library of Congress Cataloging-in-Publication Data

Latino elders and the twenty-first century: issues and challenges for culturally competent research and practice / Melvin Delgado, editor.

     p. cm.

     "Co-published simultaneously as Journal of Gerontological Social Work, vol. 30, numbers 1/2 1998."

     Includes bibliographical references and index.

     ISBN 0-7890-0657-X (alk. paper)–ISBN 0-7890-1327-4 (alk. paper)

     1. Hispanic American aged–Services for. I. Delgado, Melvin.

HV1461.L37 1998

362.6′089′68073–dc21

98-51288

CIP

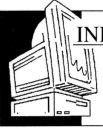

INDEXING & ABSTRACTING

Contributions to this publication are selectively indexed or abstracted in print, electronic, online, or CD-ROM version(s) of the reference tools and information services listed below. This list is current as of the copyright date of this publication. See the end of this section for additional notes.

- *Abstracts in Social Gerontology: Current Literature on Aging*

- *Academic Abstracts/CD-ROM*, EBSCO Publishing Editorial Department, P.O. Box 590, Ipswich, MA 01938-0590

- *Academic Search: data base of 2,000 selected academic serials, updated monthly*: EBSCO Publishing, P.O. Box 590, Ipswich, MA 01938-0590

- *AgeInfo CD-Rom*

- *AgeLine Database*

- *Alzheimer's Disease Education & Referral Center (ADEAR)*

- *Applied Social Sciences Index & Abstracts (ASSIA) (Online: ASSI via Data-Star) (CDRom: ASSIA Plus)*

- *Behavioral Medicine Abstracts*

- *Biosciences Information Service of Biological Abstracts (BIOSIS)*

- *Brown University Geriatric Research Application Digest "Abstracts Section"*

- *caredata CD: the social and community care database*

- *CINAHL (Cumulative Index to Nursing & Allied Health Literature), in print, also on CD-ROM from CD PLUS, EBSCO, and SilverPlatter, and online from CDP Online (formerly BRS), Data-Star, and PaperChase. (Support materials include Subject Heading List, Database Search Guide, and instructional video.)*

(continued)

- *CNPIEC Reference Guide: Chinese National Directory of Foreign Periodicals*

- *Criminal Justice Abstracts*

- *Current Contents:* Clinical Medicine/Life Sciences (CC: CM/LS) (weekly Table of Contents Service), and Social Science Citation Index. Articles also searchable through Social SciSearch, ISI's online database and in ISI's Research Alert current awareness service.

- *Expanded Academic Index*

- *Family Studies Database (online and CD/ROM),* National Information Services Corporation, 306 East Baltimore Pike, 2nd Floor, Media, PA 19063

- *Family Violence & Sexual Assault Bulletin*

- *Human Resources Abstracts (HRA)*

- *IBZ International Bibliography of Periodical Literature*

- *Index to Periodical Articles Related to Law*

- *MasterFILE: updated database from EBSCO Publishing,* P.O. Box 590, Ipswich, MA 01938-0590

- *National Clearinghouse for Primary Care Information (NCPCI)*

- *New Literature on Old Age*

- *Periodical Abstracts, Research I (general & basic reference indexing & abstracting data-base from University Microfilms International (UMI), 300 North Zeeb Road, P.O. Box 1346, Ann Arbor, MI 48106-1346)*

- *Periodical Abstracts, Research II (broad coverage indexing & abstracting data-base from University Microfilms International (UMI), 300 North Zeeb Road, P.O. Box 1346, Ann Arbor, MI 48106-1346)*

- *Psychological Abstracts (PsycINFO)*

- *Social Planning/Policy & Development Abstracts (SOPODA)*

(continued)

- *Social Science Source: coverage of 400 journals in the social sciences area; updated monthly*; EBSCO Publishing, P.O. Box 590, Ipswich, MA 01938-0590

- *Social Sciences Index (from Volume 1 & continuing)*

- *Social Work Abstracts*

- *Sociological Abstracts (SA)*

Special Bibliographic Notes related to special journal issues (separates) and indexing/abstracting:

- indexing/abstracting services in this list will also cover material in any "separate" that is co-published simultaneously with Haworth's special thematic journal issue or DocuSerial. Indexing/abstracting usually covers material at the article/chapter level.

- monographic co-editions are intended for either non-subscribers or libraries which intend to purchase a second copy for their circulating collections.

- monographic co-editions are reported to all jobbers/wholesalers/approval plans. The source journal is listed as the "series" to assist the prevention of duplicate purchasing in the same manner utilized for books-in-series.

- to facilitate user/access services all indexing/abstracting services are encouraged to utilize the co-indexing entry note indicated at the bottom of the first page of each article/chapter/contribution.

- this is intended to assist a library user of any reference tool (whether print, electronic, online, or CD-ROM) to locate the monographic version if the library has purchased this version but not a subscription to the source journal.

- individual articles/chapters in any Haworth publication are also available through the Haworth Document Delivery Service (HDDS).

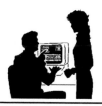

Latino Elders
and the Twenty-First Century:
Issues and Challenges
for Culturally Competent
Research and Practice

CONTENTS

ABOUT THE EDITOR

Melvin Delgado, PhD, is Professor and Chair of Macro-Practice Sequence in the School of Social Work at Boston University. He has been principal investigator on many studies funded by organizations such as the Center on Substance Abuse Prevention, the U.S. Department of Education, and the National Institutes of Health, among others. A member of the editorial boards of the *Journal of Multicultural Social Work*, *Social Work with Groups*, and *Alcoholism Treatment Quarterly*, Dr. Delgado is the author or co-author of numerous government reports, book chapters, and articles that have appeared in such journals as *Health and Social Work*, *Social Work in Education*, *Drugs & Society*, and *Social Work*. In addition, he is co-editor of the book *Social Work Approaches to Alcohol and Other Drug Problems: Case Studies and Teaching Tools for Educators and Practitioners* (Council on Social Work Education, 1997), author of *Social Work Practice in Non-Traditional Urban Settings* (Oxford University Press, 1998), and editor of *Alcohol Use/Abuse Among Latinos: Issues and Examples of Culturally Competent Services* (The Haworth Press, Inc., 1998).

Foreword

I need to express my admiration for the work Professor Melvin Delgado and his colleagues have done to make this collection an important contribution to the literature, and to urge all readers to give the articles included here a careful read.

I know that this will prove to be a very useful book in your professional library, and that you will continue to use it and refer to it in the years ahead.

I congratulate Professor Delgado and the other authors of these papers, and I take pride in this being a *Journal of Gerontological Social Work* publication.

Rose Dobrof, DSW

[Haworth co-indexing entry note]: "Foreword." Dobrof, Rose. Co-published simultaneously in *Journal of Gerontological Social Work* (The Haworth Press, Inc.) Vol. 30, No. 1/2, 1998, p. xvii; and: *Latino Elders and the Twenty-First Century: Issues and Challenges for Culturally Competent Research and Practice* (ed: Melvin Delgado) The Haworth Press, Inc., 1998, p. xv. Single or multiple copies of this article are available for a fee from The Haworth Document Delivery Service [1-800-342-9678, 9:00 a.m. - 5:00 p.m. (EST). E-mail address: getinfo@haworthpressinc.com].

Preface

The topic of this book is on Latino elders and the challenges they will present for the field of gerontology in the twenty-first century. Latino elders are increasing numerically and are projected to continue to do so well into the next century (Hayes-Bautista, Schink & Chapa, 1988; Treas, 1995). This population group, in addition, is increasing in diversity and is no longer limited to Mexican American, Puerto Rican or Cuban heritage. No geographical area of the country will escape the impact of this group.

The field of gerontological social work, research as well as practice, will encounter tremendous challenges as it attempts to meet the needs of Latino elders utilizing culturally competent principles. There are a variety of cultural factors, issues, and needs that must be understood in order to better serve Latino elders. These areas will be identified and analyzed and a set of recommendations made to help researchers, practitioners, and organizations better meet the needs of Latinos.

The focus of this collection is to work from a conceptual framework to case studies and examples. This volume consists of two sections. The first section consists of three articles delineating a conceptual framework and providing a demographic picture of Latino elders. The second section consists of eight articles that address a variety of Latino elder needs across ethnic-specific groups.

In section one, the article written by Dr. Steven Lozano Applewhite titled "Culturally Competent Practice with Elderly Latinos" provides readers with a theoretical foundation on the concept of cultural competence and the challenges of achieving it in practice with Latinos. Many gerontological organizations cannot rely solely on hiring Latino staff to ensure culturally competent services; they must, as a result, also develop mechanisms to help non-Latino staff refine their skills and knowledge on the topic. The article by Dr. Emelicia Mizio titled "Staff Development: An Ethical Imperative" addresses the needs of staff to achieve cultural competence with Latino Elders,

[Haworth co-indexing entry note]: "Preface." Delgado, Melvin. Co-published simultaneously in *Journal of Gerontological Social Work* (The Haworth Press, Inc.) Vol. 30, No. 1/2, 1998, pp. xix-xxi; and: *Latino Elders and the Twenty-First Century: Issues and Challenges for Culturally Competent Research and Practice* (ed: Melvin Delgado) The Haworth Press, Inc., 1998, pp. xvii-xix. Single or multiple copies of this article are available for a fee from The Haworth Document Delivery Service [1-800-342-9678, 9:00 a.m. - 5:00 p.m. (EST). E-mail address: getinfo@haworthpressinc.com].

xvii

and the role of staff training as a vehicle for doing so. Dr. Melvin Delgado's article "Puerto Rican Elders and Merchant Establishments: Natural Caregiving Systems or Simply Businesses?" reports on research focused on identifying community resources in service to one Latino group in a medium size New England city.

In section two, Drs. Paz and Aleman's article titled "The Yaqui Elderly of Old Pascua" raises reader consciousness of a Latino group that is very often misunderstood for being Native American in the southwest region of the country. Dr. Ana Paulino writes on Dominicans, a Latino group that is increasing numerically but has been overlooked in the professional literature. Dr. Sánchez-Ayéndez's article "Middle-Aged Puerto Rican Women as Primary Caregivers to the Elderly: A Qualitative Analysis of Everyday Dynamics" presents an ethnographic picture of Puerto Rican caregivers and provides an invaluable glimpse into the day-to-day struggles of being a primary caregiver.

Drs. Hazuda, Wood, Lichtenstein and Espino's article "Sociocultural Status, Psychosocial Factors and Cognitive Functional Limitation in Elderly Mexican Americans: Findings from the San Antonio Longitudinal Study of Aging" highlights the importance for social workers to be aware of the constellation of psychosocial resources and burdens related to the cognitive function of Mexican-American elders. Drs. Kail and DeLaRosa focus on an area rarely looked at in the professional literature, namely, the impact of alcohol, tobacco and other drugs on Latino elders, and the challenge in providing culturally competent services.

Drs. Torres-Gil and Kuo's article "Social Policy and the Politics of Hispanic Aging" examines how Latino elders, through their voting, can influence setting a national agenda that benefits them. The article by Calderón and Tennstedt titled "Ethnic Differences in the Expression of Caregiver Burden: Results of a Qualitative Study" raises the importance of understanding caregiver burden within a cultural context. Tennstedt, Chang, and Delgado's article "Patterns of Long-Term Care: A Comparison of Puerto Rican, African-American, and Non-Latino White Elders" reports on the findings of a cross-sectional study in a large New England city and draws implications for service delivery based upon ethnic/racial factors and considerations.

Melvin Delgado, PhD
Professor of Social Work
Chair of Macro-Practice
School of Social Work
Boston University
Boston, MA

REFERENCES

Hayes-Bautista, D.E., Schink, O.W. & Chapa, J. (1988). *The burden of support: Young Latinos in an aging society.* Stanford, CA: Stanford University Press.

Treas, J. (1995). Older Americans in the 1990s and beyond. *Population Bulletin, 50,* 2.

Culturally Competent Practice
with Elderly Latinos

Steven Lozano Applewhite, PhD

Cultural diversity is a concept that embraces the multiple dimensions of human identity, biculturality, and culturally defined social behaviors. In the broadest sense, it encompasses people of color, women, the aged, gays and lesbians, physically and emotionally challenged, the poor and homeless, and a host of other disenfranchised groups. Lum (1992) notes that cultural diversity has long been a cornerstone of social work education, and a blueprint for understanding human behavior in the physical, cognitive-affective-behavioral, and social environmental context. Culture and human behavior thus represent the constant and dynamic interplay between individuals and their environment. Lum adds that culturally diverse social work practice recognizes and respects a variety of populations but primarily refers to people of color, particularly Latinos, African-Americans, Asian-Americans, and Native-Americans, who have experienced historical oppression and racism, prejudice and discrimination in society.

Clearly, cultural diversity is a significant element of social work education and practice. Within this context a new field of practice has emerged from the literature with a distinct terminology, knowledge base, value orientation, skills and approaches for social work practice. Among these approaches are "ethnic sensitive practice" (Devore and Schlesinger, 1991), "cultural awareness" (Green, 1995), "process-stage social work" (Lum, 1996), "ethnic competence" (Green, 1985; Mayes, 1978), and "culturally competent practice" (Cross, 1989; Leigh, 1998). Central to these approaches is the view that

Steven Lozano Applewhite is Associate Professor, University of Houston, Houston, TX 77204-4492.

[Haworth co-indexing entry note]: "Culturally Competent Practice with Elderly Latinos." Applewhite, Steven Lozano. Co-published simultaneously in *Journal of Gerontological Social Work* (The Haworth Press, Inc.) Vol. 30, No. 1/2, 1998, pp. 1-15; and: *Latino Elders and the Twenty-First Century: Issues and Challenges for Culturally Competent Research and Practice* (ed: Melvin Delgado) The Haworth Press, Inc., 1998, pp. 1-15. Single or multiple copies of this article are available for a fee from The Haworth Document Delivery Service [1-800-342-9678, 9:00 a.m. - 5:00 p.m. (EST). E-mail address: getinfo@haworthpressinc.com].

1

culture and ethnicity are critical dimensions that are pivotal in the delivery of services to culturally diverse clients.

This chapter describes a framework for culturally competent practice with elderly Latinos. It is based on the notion that the concept of culture provides insight into the dynamics of human behavior and serves as a tool for cultural intervention. As proposed in this framework, practitioners must gain an understanding of the issues and problems facing elderly Latinos, as well as a theoretical foundation in gerontological theory, and familiarity with the principles of culturally competent social work practice, in order to integrate these concepts into their practice. Within the limits of this paper, four major components are described as building blocks for culturally competent practice with elderly Latinos. The first component provides a cursory overview of the socio-economic status of elderly Latinos, the fastest growing elderly population in this country. The second component examines the bio-psychosocial aspects of aging, focusing on the issue of cultural relevance in gerontological theories. The third component identifies the fundamental principles of culturally competent social work practice with elderly Latinos. The final component describes the ecological perspective to exemplify the relevance of culture and ethnicity in culturally competent practice with elderly Latinos.

DEMOGRAPHICS OF ELDERLY LATINOS

By the turn of the century the demographic shifts in this country will reflect an unprecedented growth in the elderly Latino population. The following figures, derived from a study of the National Council of La Raza (NCLR) (1991), present an overview of the demographic and socioeconomic status of elderly Latinos in the United States. According to NCLR the elderly Latino population which is growing at a faster rate than the non-Latino population, is estimated to reach 6.3 percent of the total elderly population by 2010. Primarily residing in the Southern and Western regions such as California (25.3%), Texas (21.2%) and Florida (13.5%), there is also a large population of Latinos in New York (10.9%). Unlike the general population, Latinos are a young population with elderly Latinos accounting for 5.2% of the total Latino population–a significant figure since the caregiving burden may fall on younger adults in the coming decade more than in previous generations. Equally significant is the fact that nearly six out of ten elderly Latinos are native-born, with Mexican Americans comprising 48 percent of the Latino population, Cuban Americans, 18 percent, Puerto Ricans, 11 percent, Central and South Americans, 8 percent, and other Latinos, 15 percent. Lamentably, this cohort of older Americans is also among the least educated elderly group in this country, with slightly over one-third with less than five years of schooling, and nearly forty percent unable to speak English.

The figures regarding income security are equally dismal with the median income for elderly Latinos being $6,642, slightly above the poverty threshold of $5,947 for individuals 65 and over. The poverty rate was estimated at 20.6 percent, twice the rate for white elderly cohorts. Health reasons and low-paying jobs have also resulted in many elderly leaving the workforce before retirement age, thereby dramatically reducing their income security and pension benefits upon retirement. Since elderly Latinos are less likely than whites and elderly African Americans to receive Social Security, or to receive private pensions or incomes from interests and other assets, there is a greater dependence on Supplementary Security Income (SSI) and public assistance programs. Ironically, elderly Latinos are least eligible to receive SSI benefits with estimates of only 44 percent of eligible Latinos receiving SSI compared to about half of the total eligible elderly population. They have greater unmet acute medical and long-term care needs, greater health problems than the general elderly population, and a history of underutilization of health and social services. Moreover, there is a misconception that elderly Latinos are cared for through the extended family system–a type of cultural safety net–and therefore are less likely to turn to formal services and programs. Unfortunately, the presumed automatic guarantees of emotional, economic and social support for elderly Latinos traditionally provided by the extended family have slowly eroded over time due to such factors as mobility, acculturation, prohibitive costs, and the multiple stresses on elderly caregivers. The high rates of poverty and unemployment also render many families incapable of adequately meeting the health, social, economic and even emotional needs of elderly Latinos. These problems are compounded by cultural barriers in the service delivery system that inhibit access to services, such as insensitive service providers, language barriers, a history of neglect, and discrimination. Combined, these statistics and trends suggest a need for a culturally competent system of service delivery that is sensitive, accessible, affordable and culturally relevant. In this context, gerontological social workers will be called upon to plan and deliver services to elderly Latinos efficiently and effectively in a culturally competent manner. To this end, culturally competent gerontological social work should begin with an understanding of the dominant theories in gerontology that underlie social work practice, and the cultural relevance of these theories to elderly Latinos.

THEORETICAL PERSPECTIVES

A starting point for culturally competent practice begins with an understanding of three broad fields of study known as the sociology, biology and psychology of aging which represent the foundation for gerontological social work practice. Of considerable value in this knowledge base is the Handbook of Aging Series which includes the *Handbook of Aging and the Social Sciences* (Binstock & George, 1990), the *Handbook of Biology of Aging* (Schneider & Rowe, 1990), and the *Handbook of the Psychology of Aging* (Birren & Schaie, 1990). However, questions abound regarding the nature and relevance of many theories of aging to elderly Latinos and people of color. The following section explores the notion of cultural relevance in three fields of aging, but is not intended to be exhaustive.

The *sociology of aging*, also referred to as the non-physical aspects of aging, focuses on the social forces and theories of aging (Atchley, 1991, p. 3). These forces include such areas as work, retirement and leisure, living environments, health care, social support systems, and others. While ethnic aging, also referred to as minority aging or ethnogerontology, was recognized as a significant area in gerontology since the early 1970s (Kent, 1971), researchers and service providers failed to treat sufficiently the substantive issues and problems facing this sub-population (Rey, 1982). Consequently, the dominant culture paradigm resulted in multiple theories of aging that are limited in relevance to elderly Latinos. Thus a fundamental concern in ethnogerontology is the extent to which aging theories and research adequately address the multiple dimensions of culture, race and ethnicity, and the impact that these factors have on social work practice with elderly Latinos. In this framework, social workers are called upon to develop a strong grasp of the dominant theories in aging with careful attention to the issue of cultural relevance with elderly Latinos. For example, do the primary concepts and underlying assumptions that guide dominant theories in aging hold true for elderly Latinos when mediated by culture and ethnicity? And to what extent have gerontological theories and strategies of intervention incorporated the unique life experiences and social conditions of elderly Latinos and other ethnic populations?

Applewhite (1997), Marin, and Marin (1991), and Stanford and Yee (1991) note that traditional empirical methods and assumptions underlying gerontology and social science research and are inadequate and often biased against elderly Latinos and other people of color. Others argue that much that passes as general theories in gerontology are more typically theoretical orientations than formal theories per se, lacking cross-cultural validity, generalizability and relevance to elderly minorities (Gibson, 1988; McNeely & Colen, 1983; Stanford & Yee, 1991). Conversely, some scholars contend that minority based research with its emphasis on socially disadvantaged populations is a narrow view, too exclusive, that overlooks the experiences and contributions of elderly white ethnic cohorts (Gibson, 1988; Weg, 1988). This view corresponds with the argument that the disadvantaged status of elderly Latinos and other minorities is a function of social class differences and not directly related to ethnicity, race and cultural differences (Markides, 1983).

Thus the difficult task of determining the relevance of such factors as ethnicity and culture advanced in the early 1970s by Dowd and Bengtson (1979) and Kent (1971) persist today in gerontology. Clearly, culturally competent practice with elderly Latinos takes greater meaning in social gerontology when the theoretical foundation, which forms the basis for practice intervention, is understood with its strengths and its limitations.

Similarly, the *biology of aging* is dominated by such theories as wear and tear, rate of living, waste product accumulation, cross-linking, free radical, and immune systems dysfunction, as well as the anatomical and physiological systems changes of old age and senescence. Senescent deterioration and life span are viewed as an inherited species-specific process. Thus the process of aging is viewed as a function of genetics, human deterioration, and environmental influences on individuals–an inescapable process common to all humans irrespective of race or ethnicity. However, the search for the universal characteristics of aging common to all humans and inescapable must be tempered with the view that the aging process varies across the human spectrum with some aspects of aging never experienced by some individuals (Cox, 1984). Sokolovosky (1997) and others raise questions about the extent to which longevity is influenced by culture and cultural variations; whether senescence is an inherited biological process; and whether there are ethnic or racial phenomena such as the "crossover effect"(Jackson, 1980) or the "double jeopardy hypothesis" (Bengtson, 1979) that explain differentials in life expectancy and life chances. Although aging is inevitable, and people experience similar patterns and problems of aging irrespective of ethnicity and culture, there are also wide-spread differences in aging patterns between elderly Latinos and the general aging population. For example, older Latinos are in poorer health than the general elderly population, with higher incidence and prevalence of chronic diseases, and a lower life expectancy than their white counterparts. These differentials demand a comprehensive understanding of the underlying causes, and the bio-physiological aspects of aging across cultures. A culturally competent practitioner will gain valuable knowledge and proficiency in practice by examining the differential patterns of aging, and cultural responses to ethnic aging.

The third field, the *psychology of aging*, is also an expansive field that includes such diverse areas as personality development, perceptual and sensory functioning, and intelligence functioning. This field was initially preoccupied with the psychology of childhood and adolescence based largely on Freudian theory. The life cycle perspective later emerged as a major area of study focusing on the developmental periods or stages of life and the corresponding tasks and life structures that start in early infancy and extend through old age. With few exceptions, stage theories failed to incorporate cultural perspective in their theories. Indeed, Troll (1982, p. 15) states that while theories vary widely, stage theories mostly assumed that people go through life in the same way (universality), through stages in the same order (sequentially), with a predetermined end point to the sequence (teleology), with a right and wrong orientation to the sequence (adaptation), and where the good is in tune with the current middle class values (class bias). Given such assumptions, it is understandable that the life experiences and life tasks of elderly Latinos remain obscure in the literature, perhaps suggesting a need for a new principle of stage development that affirms culture and ethnicity as powerful determinants of human development (cultural relevance).

Fortunately, in the last decade the life span developmental perspective has witnessed considerable growth, focusing on the biological, social, and psychological factors in human development, with less attention to chronological age as an explanatory variable (Kart, 1994, p. 156). Accordingly, Germain (1991) recommends a reconsideration of the stage model of individual development to emphasize the impact of *ethnicity* (emphasis added) on the life course and "the unique paths of development people take in varied environments, as well as their varied life experiences from birth to old age" (Devore & Schlesinger, 1996, p. 77). Similarly, Gibson (1988) contends that the study of elders of color is more appropriately served by focusing on a life course perspective and "the interrelatedness of changing social structures, social-historical periods, personal biographies, life cycle stages, personal adaptive resources, life events and well being as integral to the study of minorities as they age" (p. 559).

Ostensibly, the psychology of aging, like other fields of gerontology, is undergoing a new stage of development, with ethnic and cultural dimensions emerging as significant factors in all areas of gerontology. This framework affirms the value of existing theories that serve as a foundation for gerontological social work practice, and assumes that the value of any gerontological theory lies in its utility and cultural relevance to diverse populations. Beyond these theories, however, gerontological social work must be grounded in the core principles and standards of social work practice.

PRINCIPLES OF CULTURALLY COMPETENT SOCIAL WORK

According to Leigh (1998), a culturally competent social worker "is aware that any helping situation must be consistent and consonant with the historical and contemporary culture of the person, family, and community. [And] take into account the nature of exchange relationships which characterize and give objective and subjective meanings to helping encounters" (p. 173). Anderson, Richardson and Leigh (1998) add seven principles for the culturally competent social worker that include: an awareness that there is much to learn about other cultures; an appreciation of regional and geographical factors and differences in cultures; a learning style based on a *person in the situation* orientation; a capacity to form relationships across cultures in social work and with other professionals; an awareness and desire to reduce power differentials between workers and clients; an ability to obtain culturally relevant information; and an ability to engage in mutual exploration, assessment and treatment of culturally diverse clients (p. 173).

For gerontological social workers, the process of becoming culturally competent is initiated through the mission and purpose of social work and operationalized through the values, knowledge and skills of the profession. In this section, these three areas are examined and adapted to reflect culturally competent practice with elderly Latinos.

Values

As noted in the *NASW Code of Ethics*, the core values of social work practice include service, social justice, dignity and worth of the person, importance of human relationships, integrity, and competence. Within these values are the ethical principles that social workers aspire to attain. Two principles that are particularly noteworthy affirm the *dignity and worth of the person,* with attention to individual, cultural and ethnic differences, and *social justice,* which sensitivity and knowledge about oppression, and cultural and ethnic diversity. Similarly, the *NASW Ethical Standards* that guide social work responsibilities emphasize *Cultural Competence and Social Diversity* in practice.

In this framework, social workers are called upon to affirm these principles and standards. Beyond these core principles, the following core values derived from the current literature on culturally competent practice (see Cross, 1989; Green, 1995; Lum, 1996; and Leigh, 1998) are adapted for practice with elderly Latinos:

- Value cultural diversity and cultural integrity with a genuine and open appreciation of inter and intra group differences among elderly Latinos.
- Value the social and historical contributions of elderly Latinos to their culture, community, and the broader society.
- Respect the help-seeking behaviors of elderly Latinos.
- Value the cultural resources and natural support system utilized by elderly Latinos in problem-solving.
- Value the strength of the nuclear and extended family and fictive kin, and the role that elder Latinos assume in this family constellation.
- Respect the traditional beliefs, folk methods, and spiritual roles of elderly Latinos in the folk healing process.
- Value culture and ethnicity as interactive and emergent forces in later life among elderly Latino cohorts.

- Validate the experiences, both positive and negative, of elderly Latinos from a social, cultural, historical, political, and spiritual perspective.

While not exhaustive, this value base provides social workers a starting point for examining their value orientation in relation to elderly Latinos, their families and communities in order to function with a greater degree of confidence and proficiency.

Knowledge

Social work knowledge is based on a range of perspectives and content areas derived from various schools of thought. Hepworth, Looney and Larsen (1997) note that the Council on Social Work Education (CSWE) categorized the knowledge base for social work practice into five content areas: Human Behavior and the Social Environment; Social Welfare Policy and Services; Social Work Practice; Research; and Practicum. The National Association of Social Workers further identified 25 knowledge areas needed for effective social work practice.

To become culturally competent, social workers must acquire technical and substantive knowledge in social work as well as cultural information about elderly Latinos in the major content areas. Berger, Federico, and McBreen, 1991; Cross et al. (1989), Devore and Schlesinger (1996), Green, (1995), Leigh (1998), Lum (1994), and Wilson (1982) identified over 50 knowledge areas and attributes essential in developing cultural and ethnic competence. These include, but are not limited, to the following:

- Knowledge about human behavior including individual and family life course considerations of elderly Latinos, and the effect that bio-psycho-social, cultural and spiritual systems have on their behavior
- Knowledge about Latino sub-cultures and elderly immigrants in particular.
- Knowledge about the impact of class, ethnicity and biculturalism on elderly Latinos.
- Knowledge about the help-seeking behaviors of elderly Latino clients.
- Knowledge about language preference, dialects, and speech and communication patterns of elderly Latinos.
- Knowledge about the perceived effectiveness of service providers and social services in meeting identifiable needs of elderly Latinos.
- Knowledge about the ways that professional values, knowledge and skills may clash with those of elderly Latinos in a helping relationship.

Clearly, the extent to which social workers increase their competency in working with elderly Latinos depends on the depth of their knowledge about

Latino cultures and their commitment to learning about diverse cultures. However, cultural knowledge does not make one culturally competent. For competency to develop, social workers must embrace a commitment of time and effort to learn about culturally diverse groups, a process that requires immersion in different cultures, and skill development in basic, intermediate and advanced techniques. The following area focuses on some culturally specific skills that may be helpful for practice with elderly Latinos.

Skills

While there are different core skills required for social work practice, McMahon (1996) categorizes foundation skills into four areas: relationship skills, problem-solving skills, political skills, and professional skills subsumed under the overarching *person in environment* perspective. The methods of practice include micro or direct practice with individuals, families and groups, and macro practice with communities, organizations, and policy and planning arenas. NASW also identified 26 skills and abilities essential for social work practice. In all, social work skills reflect a broad range of interpersonal, technical, therapeutic and organizational skills that are comprehensive, complex and enable social workers to work with diverse populations and settings.

Culturally competent practice builds on foundation skills in social work practice as exemplified by Leigh (1998), Mayes (1978), Wilson (1982) and others who identified specific skills for culturally competent social work practice. The following represent a cross section of such proposed skills adapted for practice with elderly Latinos:

- Ability to communicate in Spanish or dialect common to elderly Latinos.
- Ability to advocate on behalf of elderly Latinos within and outside their communities.
- Ability to recognize racial and ethnic biases and issues in organizations and practice settings, and to confront racism and discrimination directed toward elderly Latinos.
- Ability to make cultural assessments on the influence of ethnicity on elderly Latinos.
- Ability to operationalize the concept of empowerment with and on behalf of elderly Latinos.
- Ability to evaluate and develop new knowledge areas, methods, and skills that are culturally appropriate for practice with elderly Latinos.
- Ability to identify the cultural coping capacity of elderly Latinos to deal with problems associated with intrapersonal, interpsychic, social structural and power relationships.

The skills that relate to this framework focus largely on the cultural dimension and cultural communication for culturally competent practice with elderly Latinos. They exemplify skills that may be acquired experientially or through formal education and training.

CULTURAL COMPETENCE
AND THE ECOLOGICAL PERSPECTIVE

The knowledge, values and skills proposed in this framework only serve as a foundation for cultural intervention with elderly Latinos. Indeed, culturally competent practice is a personal and professional matter, one which requires each professional to embrace the concept of cultural diversity and to develop a practice framework that reflects their level of experience, comfort and familiarity. In this framework, the ecological perspective is suggested as one approach that is considered uniquely suited for practice with elderly Latinos. It provides a contextual framework for understanding how elderly Latinos interact in later life within a biopsychosocial, cultural and spiritual context. This perspective reflects the integration of gerontological theories and human development across the life cycle, emphasizing the reciprocal interaction that occurs between the person and their environment, and the influence that culture and ethnicity have on elderly Latinos across the macro, meso and micro levels (Bronfenbrenner, 1979; Germain, 1979; Germain & Gitterman, 1980). At each systemic level, elderly Latinos are engaged in a set of *transactions* or reciprocal exchanges with their environment, both *adaptive* and *maladaptive*, that influence their ability to interact in a mutually responsive manner in search of a *goodness of fit*, matching the elderly Latinos needs with the resources in their immediate environment. This perspective views the elderly's physical and social settings as the most appropriate situations for understanding the forces that shape human behavior and development. It recognizes that elderly Latinos are *goal directed* and *purposeful*, seeking *relatedness* to significant others through social, emotional and cultural exchanges, and constantly striving for *competence* and self confidence in their judgments, decisions and relationships (Greene & Ephross, 1991). Key concepts such as *transactions, goodness of fit, relatedness,* and *competence* are significant in this perspective; however, none may be as relevant to elderly Latinos as the concepts of *culture* and *ethnicity*.

As discussed in this framework, *culture* represents a way of life that binds elderly Latinos together through their culture, language, nationality, values, beliefs and practices that are considered appropriate and desirable. It guides and influences their thinking and shapes their behavior in the social environment (Berger, Federico, & McBreen, 1991; Greene & Ephross, 1991). Broadly defined, culture is a way of life and the way people guide and structure their behavior. Berger, Federico, and McBreen (1991) note that "Culture represents humankind's master plan; it molds our way of explaining the world and charts the limits of allowable behavior" (p. 30). Combined, these elements of culture provide a blueprint for understanding behavior, and how elderly Latinos define and give "meaning" to their lives developmentally. However, culture is more than a worldview, a set of patterns, activities, symbols, rituals or language. Culture is a "problem-solving device and technical tool that facilitates the helping process"(Leigh, 1998, p. 30).

Ethnicity is an equally significant concept in the ecological perspective with multiple definitions and relevance to service providers. In the broadest sense, ethnicity refers to a sense of peoplehood, a psychological and social identity involving commonality and loyalty to race, religion, nationality and ancestry (Cox & Ephross, 1998; Devore and Schlesinger, 1996). It is distinguishable as categorical and transactional ethnicity (Green, 1995). Categorical ethnicity refers to specific predetermined traits or "content" about a group such as color, food, music, dress, and the like, believed to be descriptive and characteristic of a particular group. In contrast, transactional ethnicity focuses more on ethnic boundaries that define a group–the manner in which people behave, communicate and act upon their differences. The former is presumed to stigmatize and perpetuate existing stereotypes and preconceived notions about ethnic groups, while the latter views ethnicity as an emergent, positive feature of human development (Green, 1995). Similarly, the concept of cultural distinctiveness (Trela & Sokolovosky, 1977) is pivotal in the ecosystem perspective. It refers to the degree to which an ethnic group is distinct in relation to their cultural values, norms and social patterns, and display high, moderate or low levels of attachment to their ancestral culture (Trela & Sokolovosky, 1977). For example many elderly Latinos embrace the Spanish language, and reserve the right to speak only Spanish. For these elderly, their language and culture are part of their identity system, providing a sense of continuity across generations, and helping them maintain a strong attachment to their ancestral culture. Their strong affinity to their culture reflects a high level of ethnic distinctiveness. In contrast, a bilingual-bicultural elderly Latino who is proficient in two languages and interacts in two cultures but does not closely adhere to either culture may reflect a moderate level of distinctiveness. An assimilated, dominant English-speaking elderly Latino with a preference for the dominant culture and little attachment to their ancestral cultures may reflect a low level of ethnic distinctiveness. This distinctiveness may be helpful in understanding an elderly's preferences, but may have limited utility in assessing the elderly's life circumstances and confronting issues. While this concept is more complex than this cursory explanation, its significance lies in its utility in helping social workers discern intragroup differences, and dispelling "myth" conceptions about elderly Latinos and people of color.

Culture and ethnicity thus serve as insulating forces in the nurturing environment for elderly Latinos and other minorities. They insulate the elderly from social and cultural affronts from the broader society, and facilitate a *goodness of fit* for the elderly and their immediate surroundings. In the nurturing environment, which may include their *communidad* and *familia*, elderly Latinos experience a high measure of *competence* and *adaptability*. They may experience high levels of *relatedness*–a desirable level of social interaction and involvement with family and friends–that is commonly absent outside their community. In cultural terms, elderly Latinos often experience a sense of belonging, purpose and *orgullo y dignidad* (pride and dignity) in the *communidad* or *barrio* (community or neighborhood), and draw their strength and support from *la cultura* (culture), *la familia* (family), *los vecinos* (neighbors), *los amistades (friends), las comadres y los compadres (fictive kin), su religion (their religion), la iglesia* (church), and a host of other natural support systems and community resources. Their level of confidence, self-esteem and pride is often heightened through positive interaction with significant others, and affirmed through their roles in the extended families and the community. Clearly, culture and ethnicity are significant forces in an eco-system perspective with profound implications for culturally competent practice with elderly Latinos.

For practitioners, knowledge and skills, coupled with a working experience and familiarity with elderly Latinos and their culture, represent building blocks for basic, intermediate or advanced levels of intervention. Culturally competent social work must be carried out in the context of micro practice with individual, families and groups, or macro practice in communities, organizations and policy arenas. Culturally competent practice in micro settings will require a redefinition of problems, needs and issues, and cultural factors that intervene in an elderly person's life. It will necessitate a reformulation of assessment and treatment strategies to incorporate the subjective dimensions of ethnicity and distinctiveness. Basic skills in exploring, assessing, contracting and evaluating necessitate effective language skills to communicate effectively with elderly Latinos. It requires an understanding of culturally specific problem-solving strategies used by the elderly in identifying and ameliorating their problems. Trust-building, establishing authentic rapport, and promoting self-esteem with elderly Latinos represent fundamental aspects of social work practice, but are critical factors for elderly Latinos who are often fearful, suspecting, indifferent, or pessimistic about social services and service providers.

Similarly, macro practice will require an understanding of the dynamics of community life, the contributions of mainstream and ethnic agencies, and the role that elderly Latinos assume in their communities. Community practice must engage the service provider and the elderly Latino in a mutual process of intervention at all levels, including problem identification, assessment, planning, goals setting, and implementation. Macro practice should provide the elderly with an opportunity to serve as cultural guides and mentors, and to empower elderly clients through the process of self-determination and self-help–fundamental principles of social work practice. The process of initiating community or organizational change must relate to the issues and constraints of ethnic communities and agencies, including identifiable strengths and weaknesses, indigenous community leadership, community and organizational readiness for change, and the role that elderly Latinos assume in the change effort.

The framework proposed in this chapter is a starting point. It is not an end in itself but a guide for engaging in a cultural learning process. It raises issues of relevance, application, principles and alternatives. It proposes a process of continuous learning–a commitment to valuing cultural diversity in its many forms and structures. It requires weeding out biases and faulty assumptions about elderly Latinos and replacing them with cultural strengths. The compelling reason for developing cultural competence is based on the notion that all elderly consumers are entitled to the most effective, responsive and sensitive treatment or service. In this regard, social workers are called upon to serve all clients equitably, to enhance human dignity and well-being, and to meet the basic human needs of the vulnerable, oppressed and impoverished in our society. As culturally competent practice evolves in the profession, gerontological social workers will respond with new and creative approaches to practice, a renewed awareness and sensitivity, and a firm commitment to valuing cultural diversity.

REFERENCES

Applewhite, S. (Nov 1995). *Curanderismo:* Demystifying the health beliefs and practices of elderly Mexican Americans. *Health and Social Work,* 20(4), 247-253.

Applewhite, S. (Jan-Feb, 1997). Qualitative research in educational gerontology. *Educational Gerontology,* 23(1), 15-27.

Atchley, R. C. (1991). *Social forces and aging* (6th ed.). Belmont, CA: Wadsworth.

Atkinson, D., Morten, G., & Sue, D.W. (1989). *Counseling American minorities.* Dubuque, IA: William C. Brown.

Bengtson, V.L. (1979). Ethnicity and aging: problems and issues in current social science inquiry. In D. Gelfand & A.J. Kutzik (Eds.) *Ethnicity and aging: Theory, research, and policy* (9-31). New York: Springer

Binstock, R., & George, L.K. (1990). *Handbook of aging and the social sciences,* 3rd ed. San Diego, CA: Academic Press.

Birren, J., & Schaie, W. (1990). *Handbook of the psychology of aging,* 3rd ed. San Diego, CA: Academic Press.

Council on Social Work Education (CSWE). (1992). *Handbook of accreditation standards and procedure* (4th ed.). Alexandria, VA: Author.

Cross, T., Bazron, B.J., Dennis, K. W., & Isaacs, M.R.(1989). *Towards a culturally competent systems of care.* Washington, DC: Georgetown University Child Development Center.

Devore, W., & Schlesinger, E.F. (1996) (4th ed.). *Ethnic-sensitive-social work practice.* Boston: Allyn & Bacon.

Dowd, J. J., & Bengtson, V. L. (1978). Aging in minority populations: An examination of the double jeopardy hypothesis. *Journal of Gerontology,* 33(3), 427-436.

Germain, C., & Gitterman, A. (1980). *The life model of social work practice.* New York: Columbia.

Germain, C.B. (1991). *Human behavior in the social environment: An ecological view.* New York: Columbia University Press.

Gibson, R.C. (1989). Minority aging research: Opportunity and challenge. *The Gerontologist* 28(4): 559-61.

Green, J. (1995). *Cultural awareness in the human services.* Boston: Allyn & Bacon.

Greene, R.R., & Ephross, P.H. (1991). *Human behavior theory and social work practice.* New York: Aldine De Gruyter.

Havighurst, R. (1968). Personality and patterns of aging. *The Gerontologist,* 8, 20-23.

Hooyman, N. & Asuman, K.H. (1993). *Social gerontology* (3rd ed.). Boston: Allyn & Bacon.

Hepworth, D. H., Rooney, R.H., & Larsen, J.A. (1997). *Direct social work practice: theory and skills.* (5th ed.). Boston: Brooks/Cole.

Jackson, J. J. (1977). *Minorities and aging.* Belmont, CA: Wadsworth.

Kart, C. S. (1994). *The realities of aging: An introduction to gerontology* (4th ed.). Boston: Allyn and Bacon.

Kent, D. (1971). The elderly in minority groups: Variant patterns of aging. *The Gerontologist,* 11, 26-29.

Leigh, J.W. (1998). *Communicating for cultural differences.* Needham Heights, MA: Allyn & Bacon.

Lum, D. (1996). *Social work practice and people of color: A process stage approach,* (3rd ed.). Boston: Brooks/Cole.

Marin, G., & Marin, B. (1991). *Research with Hispanic populations.* Newbury Park, CA: Sage.

Markides, K. S. (1983). Minority aging. In M. W. Riley, B.B. Hess, & K. Bond (Eds.), *Aging and society: Selected reviews of recent research* (pp. 115-138). Hillsdale, NJ: Lawrence Erlbaum Associates.

Markides, K.S., & Mindel, C.H. (1987). *Aging and ethnicity.* Beverly Hills, CA: Sage.

McNeely, R. L., & Colen, J.N. (1983). Minority aging and knowledge in the social professions: Overview of a problem. In R. J. McNeely & J.N. Cohen (Eds.) *Aging in minority groups* (pp 15-23). Beverly Hills, CA: Sage.

National Association of Social Workers (1996). *Code of ethics of the National Association of Social Workers.* Silver Springs, MD: NASW Press.

National Council of La Raza (February, 1991). Being involved in the aging network:

A planning and resource guide for Hispanic community-based organizations. Policy Analysis Center and Office of Institutional Development. Washington, D.C.

Neugarten, B.L. (1968). Adult personality: Toward a psychology of the life cycle. In B.L. Neugarten (Ed.), *Middle age and aging* (pp. 137-147). Chicago: University of Chicago Press.

Norton, D. G. (1978). *The dual perspective.* New York: Council on Social Work Education.

Schneider, E. L., & Rowe, J.W. (1990). *Handbook of the biology,* 3rd ed. San Diego, CA: Academic Press.

Sohng, S., & Ashford, J.B. (1994). Are traditional empirical research methods inherently biased against people of color? In W.W. Hudson and P.S. Nurius (Eds.), *Controversial issues in social work research* (pp. 22-36). Thousand Oaks, CA: Sage.

Sokolovosky, J. (1990). *The cultural context of aging.* New York: Bergin and Garvey.

Solomon, B. (1976). *Black empowerment: Social work in oppressed communities.* New York: Columbia.

Stanford, E. P., & Yee, D.L. (1991). Gerontology and the relevance of diversity. *Generations,* 15(4), 11-14.

Sue, D.W., & Sue, D. (1990). *Counseling the culturally different.* New York: John Wiley.

Thomae (1980). Personality development in adulthood and old age. In J.E. Birren & R.B. Sloane (Eds.), *Handbook of mental health and aging.* Englewood Cliffs, NJ: Prentice-Hall.

Troll, L.E. (1982). *Continuations: Adult development and aging.* Monterey, CA: Brooks/Cole.

Weg, R.B. (1988, October/November). The impact of human diversity on curricula for gerontology. *AGHE Exchange Newsletter,* 12(1), 1-3.

Staff Development:
An Ethical Imperative

Emelicia Mizio, DSW

This article will address staff development issues with reference to cultural competency, focused on the Hispanic elderly. It will be important to keep in mind "that there is a central core of values, knowledge, and skill that undergrids work with all groups. As social workers we have at minimum a general, philosophical, theoretical, and practice base from which we can build to work with minority populations" (Mizio, 1981). This core will be the foundation upon which staff development will proceed.

Practitioners who believe that social workers can effectively work with all groups without applying cultural modifications, and those who do not recognize the commonalities in practice with all human beings irrespective of race, ethnicity, and gender, will do a disservice to their clients, negating either their humanity or uniqueness. "Ignoring the importance of ethnicity may harm the lives of many older individuals. Overstating the importance of ethnicity may also be damaging" (Gelfand & Barresi, 1987). There are common human needs that are expressed through cultural filters and which need to be responded to in working with diverse elderly client populations. It is necessary for staff developers to keep this perspective in their work with practitioners.

Culturally competent practice targeted to the Hispanic elderly can be enhanced by staff development programs that are understood by each agency to be only a small part of the total organization's commitment to and investment in quality practice. Staff development programs are critically necessary to reach a higher standard of service delivery to Latino seniors than is currently in existence.

Emelicia Mizio is Chairperson, Department of Social Work, Indiana State University, Terre Haute, IN 47809.

[Haworth co-indexing entry note]: "Staff Development: An Ethical Imperative." Mizio, Emelicia. Co-published simultaneously in *Journal of Gerontological Social Work* (The Haworth Press, Inc.) Vol. 30, No. 1/2, 1998, pp. 17-32; and: *Latino Elders and the Twenty-First Century: Issues and Challenges for Culturally Competent Research and Practice* (ed: Melvin Delgado) The Haworth Press, Inc., 1998, pp. 17-32. Single or multiple copies of this article are available for a fee from The Haworth Document Delivery Service [1-800-342-9678, 9:00 a.m. - 5:00 p.m. (EST). E-mail address: getinfo@haworthpressinc.com].

17

STAFF DEVELOPMENT DEFINED

Staff development, according to the *Social Work Dictionary* (Barker, 1995) refers to, "Activities and programs within an organization designed to enhance the abilities of personnel to fulfill the existing and changing requirements of their job." A whole array of activities are listed, which include short-term in-service training classes as well as funding for attending training and meetings outside the agency. Outside speakers and consultants, group conferences, and provision of information are also strategies enumerated.

Staff development is noted to have a broader function, that of assisting personnel with improving career objectives and opportunities. It also is described as serving the latent purpose of recruitment and retention of competent personnel, and "humanizing" the agency (Barker, 1995). In-service training, central to staff development programs, is defined in terms of productivity and efficiency as related to organizational objectives. Supervisors and consultants provide that function (Barker, 1995).

If an organization is to achieve cultural competency, its staff development program, with its component of in-service training, would best be reconceptualized to highlight its ultimate purpose, that being the delivery of quality services responsive to clients' and potential service consumers' definitions of needs and solutions.

STAFF DEVELOPMENT AND CULTURE

Staff development efforts will need to reflect on the organization's, worker's, and client's world view and help to determine their practice implications. Consider that even when speaking the same language, people from different cultures "tend to have different definitions for the same nonverbal and verbal messages" (Witte & Morrison, 1995).

The manner in which difficulties are defined has strong cultural components. The Hispanic elderly have their own framework for interpreting their problems and will diagnose and label them in their own particular manner. Health issues, for example, are an important concern. A key aspect to one's world view is the ethnomedical system, the way in which a culture's member perceives health and disease. It is essential to learn to what extent the Hispanic elderly client subscribes to a personalistic, naturalistic, or Western (scientific) view. At the very least it will effect medication compliance.

In staff development efforts social workers will need to be taught how to reach for meanings in themselves and clients and to intervene using labels, terms, and concepts that the Hispanic elderly can understand in health and other areas. It is the worker who is required to "frame health–and disease related messages within . . . [the client's] world view . . . and develop messages that the patient or audience can understand" (Witt & Morrison, 1995). For evaluation of outcomes, the Hispanic elderly's values and expectations are imperative "because treatment can be considered successful only if the elderly Hispanic client or the Hispanic community view it as such" (Gallegos, 1991).

CULTURAL COMPETENCY

The Council on Social Work Education (CSWE) and the National Association of Social Workers (NASW) in their leadership roles are concerned with the profession educating social workers who, in their practice, meet the requirements of a culturally pluralistic society and who are able to serve populations at risk. One such vulnerable group is the Hispanic elderly population with its double jeopardy status. This term is not being used to mean widening ethnic differentials with age or worsening family relationships (Markides, 1987). It is rather to take note that "The affects of unequal opportunity, spawned by discrimination, are too readily apparent in the current status and disadvantaged living conditions of many minority elderly persons today" (Gould, 1989). Social work has yet to develop the personnel to effectively educate students as culturally competent social workers, who in turn can serve as a work pool to build up the capacity to serve effectively such groups at risk.

NASW in its policy document, *Social Work Speaks* (1997), states "Social workers have an ethical responsibility to be culturally competent practitioners, as the NASW Code of Ethics (1996) suggests." Fulfillment of this ethical responsibility demands a requisite value, knowledge, and skill base.

The policy document (NASW, 1997) defines cultural competence as "a set of congruent behaviors, attitudes, and policies that come together in a system or agency or among professionals and enable the system, agency, or professionals to work effectively in cross-cultural situations." This implies the need for total agency involvement at all levels in the process of insuring a competent agency and competent professionals in the delivery of culturally responsive services to all clients.

THE ORGANIZATIONAL CONTEXT
FOR STAFF DEVELOPMENT

Staff development efforts take place in an organizational context, which in turn takes place in a societal one. Organizations, like individuals, groups, and society, possess cultures. The organizational culture is reflective of the societal culture. Organizations are linked to the stage of development of a particular society (Morgan, 1986). American society has yet to come to terms with its multicultural population. The English Only movement demonstrates its conflict.

Schriver (1995) examines the manner in which societal paradigms have shaped theories and practice in social work. The dominant or traditional paradigm, the world view that shapes our society, is Eureocentric. This perspective, therefore, influences us as individuals, impacts us as social workers, and helps shape the institutions in which we practice. "What this has come to mean is that all persons, both white and non-white, have come to be judged or evaluated in virtually all areas of life according to the standards that reflect the values, attitudes, experiences and historical perspectives of white persons, specifically white persons of European Descent" (Schriver, 1995).

The extent to which an organization is able to adopt an alternative paradigm will affect all aspects of its practice and training. The inherent dignity and worth of all individuals become the true standards for evaluation of a person's worth and importance. Respect for a client is in the context "in which the client is an active party to the definition of how that context is to be understood" (Hugman, 1996). Diversity is celebrated. There would be a recognition of how oppression has affected and is affecting the lives of the Hispanic elderly, with efforts made to eliminate the destructive conditions upon which the Hispanic elderly live.

Ferdman and Brody (1996) discuss models of diversity training in business. A distinction is made between the social diversity and social justice approaches. The social diversity approach focuses on a look at culture, how people differ, and the need to move forward. The social justice approach examines and confronts the dimension of discrimination and oppression by identifying its form, its operating and perpetuating mechanisms, and the ways in which it can be eradicated in its very own organization. Thus in human service organizations how services are structured provide a strong message. A critical question to ask is, "Do the practitioner and client systems experience the organization as being or wanting to be Hispanic elderly friendly?"

Ferdman and Brody (1996) point out that it is necessary to understand that diversity training is but one aspect of a larger set of diversity initiatives and interventions. A diversity initiative to be effective requires acknowledging that the organizational system with its policies and practices also will likely require changes. Diversity initiatives require resources and infusion at all organizational levels, for without this commitment, line level employees providing direct services will resist changing or be unable to change, kept in place by the system and its "inflexible bureaucratic demands" (Wong & Gibbs, 1995).

The author for many years conducted cultural awareness workshops for public social service employees in eligibility sections serving an Hispanic elderly population. Participants found language barriers especially frustrating and were angered at the Hispanic elderly's difficulty in speaking English. Trainees became motivated to speak some key Spanish phrases related to the application process, and to be patient with applicants in their attempts to communicate. On their return weeks later to the second part of the workshop, the employees reported they had gotten in trouble for not being able to meet interview quotas when experimenting with new approaches.

The problems experienced demonstrate the absolute necessity for administrators and supervisors to be involved in training efforts. "The social work supervisor represents a critical professional role model for workers. The supervisor's behavior will best demonstrate what he or she hopes will be learned by the supervisee. . . . What effective supervisors 'say to do' need to be congruent with what they themselves 'do'" (Gitterman & Miller, 1977).

Role modeling in current terminology is often spoken of in terms of the parallel process, which gives consideration to how the supervisor treats the worker and the worker in turn replicates this type of behavior with clients. "More is 'caught' by staff than is 'taught' by the supervisor" (Shulman, 1995). More is duplicated by the supervisee than the manner in which she or he is treated. If the supervisor looks at the worker's client through a racist lens, wittingly or unwittingly, the racist attitudes will be picked up easily by the worker.

Even when employees demonstrated willingness to behave differently towards their Hispanic elderly clients they found themselves in a system that asked them in effect to preserve the status quo. Departmental policies placed workers in a role conflict situation. The roles of culturally competent employee, and a high producing employee were at odds, defeating the purpose and outcome of the training. "Regardless of the organization's stated aims or official goals [with its staff development training efforts], the allocation of available resources indicates what the organization intends to accomplish because these allocations manifest the preferences and choices made by those who control the organization's resources" (Davis-Sacks & Hazenfeld, 1987).

KEY ASSUMPTIONS
UNDERLYING STAFF DEVELOPMENT EFFORTS
TOWARDS CULTURAL COMPETENCY

Assumption 1. Staff development builds on the foundation of a common base of social work values, knowledge, and interventive skills.

> Full recognition of the common base will mean . . . that discussions of various aspects of social work and its practice . . . rest on and derive

their meaning from the common base of the profession . . . [which] comes first because it is the essence of the profession, and the segments all take their place in relation to the common base. (Bartlett, 1970)

Bartlett elaborated on values and concepts of helping clients to grow to their full potential, client self determination, acceptance of the client, centrality of the client-worker relationship, and worker self awareness. Interventions included a full "interventive repertoire," what we would today term multimethods and multilevels strategies directed toward improving the quality of society, and providing sufficient environmental resources to improve the social functioning of clients.

Assumption 2. Staff development may serve to reinforce social workers' commitment to the NASW Code of Ethics through providing information on the new Code (effective January 1, 1997), and its discussion in terms of an ethical imperative.

The Code provides ethical guidelines for working with all clients and is useful for work with Hispanic elderly clients. The core values specified service, social justice, dignity and worth of the person, importance of human relationships, integrity, and competence are certainly those which would be expected as a beginning point for culturally competent practice.

Assumption 3. Staff development stresses the value of the generalist practice model, even in clinical settings, and reminds workers that they have the ability to work from this model, for which current social work education attempts to prepare, and practice with the Hispanic elderly demands.

The roots of social work are founded upon the generalist model. Definitions may vary but "There appears to be a definitional agreement on the centrality of the multimethod and multilevel approaches, based on an eclectic choice of theories base and the necessity for incorporating the dual vision of the profession on private issues and social justice concerns" (Landon, 1995).

Information with reference to group demographics, history, and current social conditions of a group is vital if social workers are to relate private troubles to public issues in a comprehensive approach to practice. The Hispanic elderly, though evidencing differences with reference to their country of origin, show in whole a high poverty rate (Gallegos, 1991).

Assumption 4. Practice requires modifications in response to cultural requirements.

Many minority elderly maintain features of their early socialization, including rural life styles, culture, language and traditions (Torres-Gil, 1987). A national survey of 2,299 living Hispanic elderly found that over 60 percent were born outside of the continental United States and 40 percent came to the continental United States at 45 years of age or older (Andrews 1989). Many Hispanics born outside of the United States have lived in barrios or Spanish-speaking enclaves (Longres, 1995). These factors clearly have implications for the level of acculturation and bear a relationship to practice.

Lum (1996) presents a number of frameworks for cross-cultural awareness practice in which practitioners could be trained. Lum states "that traditional social work practice could be infused with ethnic meaning." Staff development should demonstrate how this is so, building on the core knowledge and skill base and staff's strengths. It should not be necessary for social workers to drastically change their methods. To expect such is to stimulate great resistance to any changes. With successful experiences, practitioners will experiment responsibly and, thereby, continue to expand the profession's cultural theoretical and practice knowledge.

Assumption 5. It is important for social workers to become conscious of the necessity to evaluate human behavior and social environment theories for their helpfulness in providing understanding of clients with other than mainstream backgrounds, and for their usefulness for cross-cultural practice.

There are many questions a worker would need to be alerted to ask in examination of a theory for applicability for work with diverse populations. A number of areas have been proposed by Greene (1994) that would take gender and cultural differences into account in looking at developmental transitions and mental health concerns, evaluating diverse social work practice, examining cultural bias, providing a multisystems perspective, interventions considering natural helping community networks, and assisting with an empowerment/advocacy sociopolitical environment. Facundo (1991) highlights the socio-political environment, which is used in the diagnosing and labeling of clients who have been entrapped socially and may be manifesting survival strategies, rather than mental illness.

Assumption 6. Staff development efforts must take note of the special significance of language for work with Hispanic elderly.

It would be important to know how a theory explains the significance of language usage and its meaning in the process of working with clients (Greene, 1994). "Language is at once a part of and the means of transmission in a culture. It incorporates the values, beliefs, and even the imagery of the culture as it facilitates thought and shapes the way in which persons view the world around them . . ." (Barresi, 1987). Barriers to service usage not only include insensitivity to cultural beliefs and traditions, but to language as well. As Hispanics age, language may become increasingly an issue, when children who have served as family translators leave home (Cox, 1987).

Mizio (1991), in a qualitative research study, explored the meaning of language to Hispanic elderly. She quotes one senior: "At the center of one's identity is language. Those though bilingual and claiming not to speak Spanish have lost their soul, have no identity and, thereby really speak no language. Who you are is tied up with your language, in which you express your being." Experience has shown that Hispanic elderly, when feeling threatened or stressed, may hide and not use the little English they do know. Language can be for the practitioner, as well, an emotionally loaded area. Language, thereby, serves as a barrier.

Assumption 7. This society is a racist one and social workers are implicated in the process and need to grow in self and other awareness and confront their stereotypes.

"To deliver racist-free services, each and every practitioner must be able to make an honest self appraisal. Each must acknowledge his or her own racist hang-ups and question where and how these are being reflected" (Mizio, 1981). The professional use of self rests on a foundation of self awareness and without which culturally competent practice would prove impossible. Ridley (1995) presents a comprehensive explication of the many ways in which unintentional racism enters the counseling and therapy process and suggests ways in which practitioners can confront this phenomenon.

Assumption 8. Social workers who continue to operate under the medical model must infuse their practice with a strength and empowerment perspective.

Under the medical model, emotional and behavioral difficulties are perceived by the social worker as mental illness. The assumption is made of some internal condition with some unknown causative element (Zastrow & Kirst-Ashman, 1997). The worker follows a study, diagnosis, and treatment framework and makes problem based assessments rather than ecological ones. People are labeled and become cases. "The focus on what is wrong often reveals an egregious *cynicism* about the ability of individuals to cope with life or to rehabilitate themselves" (Saleeby, 1997).

Many Hispanic elderly have lived their lives under harsh circumstances, experiencing poverty and discrimination throughout the years. Out of the 28 Hispanic seniors interviewed in the previously cited study (Mizio, 1991), over three-fourths felt discriminated against by Anglos and African Americans, a group amongst whom they often reside and with whom they share many a waiting room for services.

"Workers operating from a strengths approach are interested in building on the strengths that have helped older adults overcome previous difficult times in their lives" (Fast & Chapin, 1997). In assessment and intervention it is important to credit their survival skills, the fact that throughout their history they have coped with the most difficult discriminatory circumstances.

The Hispanic elderly's resource network can be used to strengthen service delivery efforts and calls for a "closer working relationship between formal and natural system" (Delgado, 1995). Facundo (1991) elaborates on the strengths, despite daily stressors, found in low income Puerto Rican families: ". . . the affective bonds among extended family members, the value placed on the community in providing diverse types of support to its members, and personalismo as a commonly shared character trait." Personalismo refers to turning secondary relationships into primary ones, and treating other with caring and respect. These strengths translate into available support, problem solving in one's native language and in a familiar social environment (Miranda, 1991).

Strengths can be found in the elderly themselves working together. An empowerment strategy used by the Institute for the Hispanic Elderly in New York was the development of the Hispanic Senior Action Council, which proved to that cohort that they could be an influential socio-political body; that could make a difference to their self-esteem and possibly improve the circumstances of their lives.

THE "HOW TO" OF STAFF DEVELOPMENT: BEYOND A MODEL AND COMPONENTS

Program Implementation and Assessment

How to achieve cultural competency in practice is the challenge facing an organization. Organizational cultural competency requires insuring well conceived staff development programs that are integrated into the fabric of the agency. Lapid-Bogda (1996) discusses diversity and organizational change in the workplace from a business perspective. Human services organizations also should engage in a solid organizational assessment of issues and underlying root causes before determining strategies to bring forth changes.

As a beginning assessment point, it is necessary to determine demographics with reference to the Hispanic elderly in the agency's catchment area. There are many other questions to be answered. Do Hispanics apply for services and return after the first interview? If not, why not? What knowledge and skill base is available or lacking in administration and workers to meet the specific service needs? How much do workers know about the Hispanic elderly cultures? Is there any Spanish and bicultural capability? In total, to what extent does the agency as a whole convey the message that it welcomes Hispanic elderly clients. Once an assessment is completed, goals and scope of activities must be established, along with roles and expectations of personnel. All of this is tied into resource availability and organizational priority setting.

The Model: Framework for Training Activities

The framework to be presented arises from the writer's many years of experience in designing and implementing workshops and courses for the purpose of developing cultural competency. The author's work at the Institute for the Hispanic Elderly contributed significantly to the formulation of these ideas. Irrespective, however, of organizational auspices, there are three components which are the sine qua non of staff development and education in the area of cultural competency. These include: self and other awareness; information theory; and culturally relevant practice adaptations.

The above categories are not discrete and can be expected to overlap, but are useful, nevertheless, for the development of separate modules. The structure and form in which these components are delivered may vary. In their delivery, the workshop leaders will be using approaches which range from the didactic to the experiential, and from the cognitive to the affective.

When training cannot be ongoing, greater impact is obtained from all-day sessions; defenses are harder to maintain and greater participation from the trainees can be secured. It is also helpful when participants are freed from work interruptions and can concentrate on the task at hand.

Self and Other Cultural Awareness Model Component

The most important component of training, perhaps, is the reminder to trainees of the critical significance of the professional use of self, which demands first a knowledge of self. The marriage of the personal self with the professional self must occur, if the worker is to be free to act upon the obligation of acting in a responsible professional manner at all times, irrespective of the client's background.

Not knowing one's own heritage serves as a barrier to the development of culturally competent practice. The educational system tends to foster a cognitive learning style and a distancing from self (Torres & Jones, 1997). "What is imperative at this initial stage is that one must first recognize, value, and understand one's own ethnic culture before recognizing, valuing, and understanding the cultures of others" (Aponte, 1995).

Staff development activities should be designed to help workers come into contact with their values, attitudes, and behaviors. "Family Roots" is one exercise that has stood the test of time. This exercise also works well as an ice breaker and to develop group cohesiveness.

Participants in the "Family Roots" exercise are instructed to discuss their backgrounds and early years, with a greater focus on the elderly and their grandparents. They compare themselves with other neighborhood families of the past, and consider whether their individual and family lifestyle today is different from their family of origin's.

The trainer focuses the trainees on the significance of culture and its transformation in their own lives. This leads easily into connections to the culture of Hispanics and Hispanic elderly as well as to their experiences with this clientele. The importance of cultural understanding to the communication process and interviewing is highlighted. A lecturette/lecture will follow. Choices related to participants' knowledge base and time constraints will determine content and depth on concepts such as culture, ethnicity, social class, acculturation, assimilation, biculturality, etc., as tied into the Hispanic elderly.

In their interaction with peers, participants are able to experience differences and similarities as interesting and enjoyable, and are more easily able to accept that commonalities or differences by themselves neither signify superiority or inferiority, or health or illness. They will be required, in effect, to do the same when meeting with clients. To communicate effectively with clients, it is important for the worker to be able to reach for the similarities and the common goals so that the differences can become less threatening to both communicants, so that the worker and elderly client will have a basis upon which to forge an alliance (Gudykunst, 1995).

Self and other awareness, in addition, means coming to terms with our stereotypes, the manner in which we categorize groups and clients of that group. Workers require assistance with dispelling myths and stereotypes. An important goal of training efforts is to help trainees become "mindful." Mindfulness involves "(a) creation of new categories; openness to new information; awareness of more than one perspective" (Gudykunst, 1995).

As social workers are also a product of our society, the issue of stereotyping is another essential area for a training focus. Cultural diversity, too often, "serves as a code-phrase used by the dominant culture to imply inferiority, undesirability, and the need for social distancing (Holmes, 1997). The Hispanic elderly are not exempt from the views society holds of Hispanics. It is essential that as social workers we achieve ". . . conscious control of our reactions when our negative stereotypes are activated is necessary to control our prejudiced responses to strangers" (Gudykunst, 1995). Necessary, too, is the workers' recognition that clients may be stereotyping workers as well. Stereotypes will serve as a barrier to relationship building unless mitigated.

Another helpful exercise is one in which the group is asked to tell about stereotypes that they have heard used to describe their own groups. The leader helps the group to examine commonalities and differences in the stereotypes and take note of how some of these terms and/or others have been applied to the Hispanic community. Trainees are also encouraged to consider how these appellations make them feel and to discuss their experiences with discrimination. Stereotypes are then evaluated from the perspective of the manner in which they can affect an individual's identity and self esteem, impact a group's chances in life, enter into intergroup relations, and consequently the worker-client encounter. They are asked to consider what Hispanic seniors may be living through and how this might impact trust in the client-worker relationship.

The content of the exercise led easily into a lecturette/lecture/discussion on the formation and purposes of stereotyping in the psychic economy of individuals and its societal use from sociological and psychological perspectives. Technical distinctions can be drawn between racism, discrimination, and prejudice, concepts which help in understanding the environmental context of Hispanic elderly life.

To understand the Other, the Hispanic elderly, it is necessary for trainers to help workers draw commonalities at an experiential level and at the same time provide cognitive reinforcements.

Information

A current and historical view of the Hispanic communities helps in understanding the backgrounds of Hispanic elderly clients. Statistical facts help to show the need for a generalist practice approach. Historical facts assist with broadening the world view of participants. It can serve to dispel myths about American largess and the feeling of some participants that Hispanics should return to their own homeland. The conquest of the southwest, and the strategic military placement of Puerto Rico become important to a realist appraisal of American history and the Hispanic condition.

The statistical portrait reflects the outcome of societal racist practices. The significance of these figures may be understood by participants cognitively. The writer has used a powerful exercise to help students appreciate the meaning of oppression experientially.

To use the "Oppressive Community" simulation exercise, trainees are instructed that they come from the planet Jupiter, which has conquered Venus. In order to maintain power they are to design the ultimate in oppressive communities. They enjoy the process and feel creative. It is an "off target" exercise in that initially it appears to bear no connection to reality. In reporting back they find that there are historical precedents for all their innovations and a lot of which has happened in the United States. They find themselves disturbed by the recognition.

As the second part of this exercise they are asked to develop strategies to overcome the oppression. They experience how difficult it is to bring forth changes from a subjugated position. This experience is not one which they soon forget. An acknowledgment of the requirement for advocacy involvement and social change strategies is truly felt by the participants.

Depending on setting, practice implications may be drawn to the feelings of hopelessness displayed by some Hispanic clients, which though perhaps relating to environmental issues now are a mental health concern. Treatment strategies that are used with non Hispanics, such as the one promoting an internal locus of control (Newman, 1995), can be considered for applicability.

Theory and Practice Adaptations

This module will vary greatly in staff development programs. Determination of program necessitates thinking through the amount of resources in money and time to be expended. The decision should focus on the service needs of the Hispanic elderly, the complexities of the workers' roles with their learning gaps, and the organizational tasks.

The investment hopefully would be more than a one time effort where generic practice hints are presented and discussed for working with the Hispanic elderly. Practice hints would include such ideas as: be careful to observe cultural niceties by addressing the senior by his/her last name; minimize social distance by telling a little of your own background; remember that the elder will not be confrontative and you can not expect a direct no answer; and do not expect to find information quickly about elderly abuse as the elderly are protective of family. Participants could role play the use of these hints in interviewing with their clients. Participants themselves could be asked to generate their own list.

Of greater value are on-going meetings in which all workers have the opportunity to discuss staff cases of elderly Hispanic client systems. When there is no internal capability, a culturally competent consultant could be used as a group leader. Hypothetical cases if necessary may be used as a beginning point.

When workers evidence difficulty in establishing a relationship or in cultural understanding of a case, and in providing appropriate interventions, the group needs to explore such factors as racism, ethnocentrism, incongruent expectations of others, lack of appreciation of impact of social forces, and subscription to the myth of the melting pot (Neukrug, 1994). Dungee-Anderson and Beckett (1995) describe two types of communication errors which would need to be assessed. Type one errors are those caused by issues related to self awareness, and type two errors are those related to defective interpretation and application of cultural knowledge.

Theoretical underpinnings for assessment, planning, and practice interventions should also be scrutinized for cultural appropriateness as related to individual cases and for general use with Hispanic clients. Readings could be assigned and processed in staff development meetings.

CONCLUSION

The effectiveness of staff development programs can not simply be determined by evaluation of the degree to which participants obtained information and knowledge about culture, societal context, demographics, practice modifications, etc. "Training in the crosscultural setting . . . requires more than knowledge of differences; it also requires acceptances of differences" (Bhagat & Prien, 1996). Beyond the acceptance of differences, social workers serving clients, not only the Hispanic elderly, ultimately will have to come to terms with the true meaning of an empowerment practice. It will be insufficient to help clients to cope or adapt; but rather, clients should be helped to achieve power to bring forth social change, in a relationship of equality with the worker (Guttierrez, GlenMaye, & DeLois, 1995).

Success of staff development in the area of diversity initiatives are extremely difficult to measure, as it is cumulative and it will take time for the progress to be demonstrated in the practitioner's work and the organization's service to the Hispanic senior. Change should be both quantitative and qualitative. The qualitative is much harder to assess. Nevertheless, where there had been an early assessment, there is a baseline from which to measure (Lapid-Bogis, 1996).

Though an agency may have established the means for evaluating the meeting of its goals, it is a complex process. It is important for social work administration to recognize the long term nature of the investment. Given the proper organizational structural supports, cultural competency should increase over time, as workers experiment responsibly, and learn from objectifying their experiences. Feedback from Hispanic elderly clients should then prove increasingly positive and each client will then serve a multiplier effect to bring other clients to the agency. Social justice, thereby, will be served.

BIBLIOGRAPHY

Andrews, J. (1989). *Poverty and poor health among elderly Hispanic Americans: A report of the Commonwealth Fund Commission on elderly people living alone.* Baltimore, MD: Commonwealth Fund Commission.

Aponte, C. I. (1995). Cultural diversity course model: Cultural competence for content and process. *Arete, 20*(1), 46-55.

Barker, R. L. (1995). *The social work dictionary* (3rd ed.). Washington, DC: NASW.

Barresi, C. M. (1987). Ethnic aging and the life course. In D. E. Gelfand and Barresi, *Ethnic Dimensions of Aging.* New York: Springer.

Bartlett, H. M. (1970). *The common base of social work practice.* Washington, DC: NASW.

Bhagat, R. S., & Prien, K. O. (1996). Cross-cultural training in organizational contexts. In D. Landis & R. S. Bhagat (Eds), *Handbook of Intercultural training* (2nd ed.). Thousand Oaks, CA: Sage Publications.

Cox, C. (1987). Overcoming Access Problems in ethnic communities. In D. E. Gelfand & C. M. Barresi (Eds.), *Ethnic dimensions of aging.* New York: Springer Publishing.

Davis-Sacks, M. L., & Hasenfeld, Y. (1987). Organization: Context for social service delivery. In A. Minaham (Ed.), *Encyclopedia of social work* (18th ed., vol. 2, pp. 204-217). Silver Spring, MD: National Association of Social Workers.

Delgado, M. (1995). Puerto Rican elders and natural support systems: Implications for human services. *Journal of Gerontological Social Work, 24*(1/2), 115-129.

Dungee-Anderson, D., & Beckett, J. O. (1995). A process model for multicultural social work practice. *Families in Society: The Journal of Contemporary Human Services, 76*(8), 459-465.

Facundo, A. (1991). Sensitive mental health services for low-income Puerto Rican families. In M. Sotomayor (ed.), *Empowering Hispanic families: A critical issue for the '90s.* Milwaukee, WI: Family Services America.

Fast, B., & Chapin, R. (1997). The strengths model with older adults: Critical practice components. In D. Saleeby (Ed.), *The strengths perspective in social work practice* (2nd ed.). White Plains, NY: Longman.

Ferdman, B. M., & Brody, S. E. (1996). Models of diversity training. In D. Landis & R. S. Bhagat (Eds.), *Handbook of intercultural training* (2nd ed.). Thousand Oaks, CA: Sage Publications.

Fong, L. G. W., & Gibbs, J. T. (1995). Facilitating services in multicultural communities in a dominant cultural setting: An organizational perspective. *Administration in Social Work, 19*(2), 1-24.

Gallegos, J. S. (1991). Culturally relevant services for Hispanic elderly. In M. Sotomayor (ed.), *Empowering Hispanic Families: A critical issue for the '90s.* Milwaukee, WI: Family Service America.

Gelfand G., & Barresi, C. M. (1987). Current perspectives in ethnicity and aging. In D. E. Gelfand & C. M. Barres (Eds.), *Ethnic dimensions of aging.* New York: Springer Publishing.

Gitterman, A., & Miller, I. (1977). Supervisors as educators. In F. W. Kaslow & Associates. San Francisco, CA: Jossey-Bass, Inc. Publishers.

Gould, J. (1989). Preface. In *Minority elderly New Yorkers.* New York: New York State Office for the Aging.

Greene, R. R. (1994). *A diversity framework.* New York: Aldine De Gruyter.

Gudykunst, W. B. (1995). Anxiety/uncertainty management theory. In R. L. Wiseman (Ed.), *Intercultural communication theory.* Thousand Oaks, CA: Sage Publications.

Gutierrez, L., GlenMaye, L., & DeLois, K. (1995). The organizational content for empowerment practice: Implications for social work administration. *Social Work, 40*(2), 249-258.

Hugman, R. (1996). Professionalization in social work: The challenge of diversity. *International Social Work, 39,* 131-147.

Landon, P. S. (1995). Generalist and advanced generalist practice. In R. L. Edwards (Ed.), *Encyclopedia of social work,* (19th ed., vol. 2, pp. 1101-1108). Washington, DC: NASW Press.

Lapid-Bogda, G. (1996). Diversity and organizational change. In G. F. Simmons (Ed.), *Cultural Diversity: Fieldbook.* Princeton, NJ: Peterson's/Pacesetter Books.

Longres, J. F. (1995). Hispanics overview. In R. L. Edwards (Ed.), *Encyclopedia of social work* (19th ed., vol. 2, pp. 1214-1222). Washington, DC: NASW Press.

Lum, D. (1996). *Social work practice and people of color: A process stage approach* (3rd. ed.). Pacific Grove, CA: Brooks/Cole Publishing.

Markides, K. S. (1987). Minorities and aging. In G. L. Maddox, (Ed.), *Encyclopedia of aging* (pp. 449-451). New York: Springer Publishing.

Miranda, M. R. (1991). Mental health services and the Hispanic elderly. In M. Sotomayor (Ed.), *Empowering Hispanic families: A critical issue for the '90s*. Milwaukee, WI: Family Services America.

Mizio, E. (1991). *A study of intergroup relations between Black and Hispanic elderly.* Unpublished doctoral dissertation, City University of New York, New York.

Mizio, E. (1981). Training for work with minority groups. In E. Mizio & A. Delaney, (Eds.), *Training for service delivery to minority clients*. New York: Family Service Association of America.

Mizio, E. (1981). Racism and the Practitioner. In E. Mizio & A. Delaney (Eds.), *Training for service delivery to minority clients*. New York: Family Service Association of America.

Morgan, G. (1986). *Images of organizations*. Beverly Hills, CA: Sage Publications.

National Association of Social Workers (1997). *Code of ethics*. Washington, DC: NASW.

Neeman, L. (1995). Using the therapeutic relationship to promote an internal locus of control in elderly mental health clients. *Journal of Gerontological Social Work, 23*(3/4), 161-176.

Neukrug, E. S. (1994). Understanding diversity in a pluralistic world. *Journal of Intergroup Relations, XXI*(2), 3-11.

Ridley, C. R. (1995). *Overcoming unintentional racism in counseling and therapy.* Thousand Oaks, CA: Sage Publications.

Saleebey, D. (1997). Introduction: Power in the people. In D. Saleebey (Ed.), *The strengths perspective in social work practice*. White Plains, NY: Longman Publishers.

Schriver, J. (1995). *Human behavior and the social environment*. Needham Heights, MA: Allyn & Bacon.

Shulman, L. (1995). Supervision and consultation. In R. L. Edwards (Ed.), *Encyclopedia of social work* (19th ed., vol. 3, pp. 2372-2379). Washington, DC: NASW Press.

Torres, J. B., & Jones, J. M. (1997). You've got to be taught: Multicultural education for social workers. *Journal of Teaching in Social Work, 15*(1/2), 161-179.

Torres-Gil, F. (1987). Aging in an ethnic society: Policy issues for aging among minority groups. In D. F. Gelfand & M. Barresi (Eds.), *Ethnic dimensions of aging*. New York: Springer Publishing.

Witte, K., & Morrison, K. (1995). Intercultural and cross-cultural health communication: Understanding people and motivating healthy behaviors. In R. L. Wisenman (Ed.), *Intercultural communication theory*. Thousand Oaks, CA: Sage Publications.

Zastrow, C., & Kirst-Ashman, K. K. (1997). *Understanding human behavior and the social environment*. Chicago, IL: Nelson-Hall Publishers.

Puerto Rican Elders
and Merchant Establishments:
Natural Caregiving Systems
or Simply Businesses?

Melvin Delgado, PhD

SUMMARY. Puerto Rican merchant establishments cover a wide range of types; these institutions historically have played important and varied natural support roles within the community. However, the professional human service literature has generally focused on grocery stores and religious institutions, ignoring most other types. This article will focus on commercial establishments not generally addressed in the literature (clothing, gift, and furniture stores, beauty parlors, botanical shops, radio stations) and draw implications for social service delivery to elders. Data were obtained through an asset assessment of a Puerto Rican community in a New England city (Holyoke, Massachusetts). *[Article copies available for a fee from The Haworth Document Delivery Service: 1-800-342-9678. E-mail address: getinfo@haworthpressinc.com]*

Melvin Delgado is Professor of Social Work and Chair, Macro-Practice Sequence, Boston University School of Social Work, 264 Bay State Road, Boston, MA 02215.

This article was made possible through funding from the National Institute on Aging (AG11171) to the New England Research Institutes, Watertown, MA and the Center for Substance Abuse Prevention (5 H86SP02208), Rockville, MD, to the Education Development Center, Newton, MA. The author was co-principle and principle investigator on these grants.

[Haworth co-indexing entry note]: "Puerto Rican Elders and Merchant Establishments: Natural Caregiving Systems or Simply Businesses?" Delgado, Melvin. Co-published simultaneously in *Journal of Gerontological Social Work* (The Haworth Press, Inc.) Vol. 30, No. 1/2, 1998, pp. 33-45; and: *Latino Elders and the Twenty-First Century: Issues and Challenges for Culturally Competent Research and Practice* (ed: Melvin Delgado) The Haworth Press, Inc., 1998, pp. 33-45. Single or multiple copies of this article are available for a fee from The Haworth Document Delivery Service [1-800-342-9678, 9:00 a.m. - 5:00 p.m. (EST). E-mail address: getinfo@haworthpressinc.com].

33

INTRODUCTION

The decade of the 1990s has witnessed exciting developments regarding the use of natural support systems/assets/resiliency approaches for reaching undervalued communities across the United States (Eckenrode, 1991; Glugoski, Reisch & Rivera, 1994; Kretzman & Mcknight, 1993; Williams & Wright, 1992). These developments have highlighted the importance of human service organizations collaborating with indigenous community resources (Barrera & Reese, 1993; Daley & Wong, 1994; Gutierrez & Ortega, 1991; Martin & Martin, 1985; Mason, 1994; Thompson & Peebles-Wilkins, 1992). These indigenous resources, in turn, are deeply rooted in cultural traditions of caregiving and care-seeking (Ghali, 1982; Longres, 1990; Morales, 1992; Rivera, 1990), and take on greater significance when a group has been uprooted to an alien land and culture (Gutierrez, Ortega & Suarez, 1990).

The social service literature on Latino elders has also witnessed an increase in publications specifically focused on utilization of natural support systems, community development, and self-help approaches (Delgado, 1995a). However, not all indigenous resources should be automatically considered to be a part of an elder natural caregiving system. Consequently, it is very important for practitioners and gerontology agencies to develop an indepth understanding of how to identify and collaborate with natural caregiving systems (Delgado, 1994).

This article reports on an asset assessment of a Puerto Rican community located in a medium size city in New England. This assessment covered a broad range of indigenous institutions that have either been ignored or superficially addressed in the professional literature, yet have tremendous implications for outreaching to Puerto Rican and other Latino elders.

OVERVIEW OF LITERATURE

The literature highlights the importance of understanding elder Puerto Rican care-seeking patterns and the role of natural support caregiving systems in helping them meet their needs (Delgado, 1995a; De La Rosa, 1988; Garrido, 1988; Sanchez, 1987; Sanchez-Ayendez, 1988). Delgado (1995a, pp. 118-119), defines Puerto Rican elder natural support systems as: ". . . a network of individuals, with or without institutional affiliation (family/ friends, religious groups, folk healers, and community institutions). They provide assistance (instrumental, informational and expressive) on an everyday basis as well as at times of crisis, and represent a community's capacity to help itself. Natural support systems also service as a mechanism for helping Puerto Ricans maintain their cultural heritage. Support systems are accessible (logistically, psychologically, conceptually, and geographically) to all sectors of the community; the assistance provided originates from relationships (familial as well as non-familial) that extend beyond the provision of services, but also entail feelings of love, affection, respect, trust, loyalty, and mutuality. In short, natural support systems have responsibility for both giving and receiving assistance."

According to Delgado and Humm-Delgado (1982), Puerto Rican natural caregiving systems generally consist of four types: (1) family/friends/close neighbors (Carrasquillo, 1994; Garcia-Preto, 1982; Rogler & Cooney, 1984); (2) religious institutions (Caraballo, 1990; Deck & Nunez, 1982; Gaiter, 1980; Rohter, 1985a; (3) folk healing centers (Carr & Perez, 1993; Harwood, 1977); and (4) merchant/social clubs (Burros, 1990; Gonzalez, 1992; Vazquez, 1974).

There is general agreement in the professional literature that family, particularly daughters, are the primary and most significant support system for Puerto Rican elders (Bastida, 1988; Sanchez, 1986; Sanchez-Ayendez, 1989, 1992). However, these studies have not specifically explored in depth the role of non-family support systems.

According to Delgado and Rosati (pending publication), in their study of Pentecostal churches, the typical church provided at least eight services that could be classified as human service in nature: (1) financial assistance; (2) friendship for the lonely; (3) interpreter; (4) food for the hungry; (5) advice/counseling; (6) community leadership; (7) information and referral to social services; and (8) child care. Meeting the needs of elders played a prominent role in the organizing and delivery of these services.

Merchant establishments, the focus of this article, are community-based institutions that provide, for profit, products and services within a cultural context; these establishments are owned, staffed, and patronized by the community. These institutions are attractive to elders because they minimize geographical, linguistic, and cultural barriers to service utilization (Delgado, 1994).

Unfortunately, the literature on merchant establishments has primarily focused on grocery stores, known in Spanish as bodegas and cormados (Agins, 1985; Carmody, 1972; Howe, 1986; Vazquez, 1974). Botanical shops (Borrello & Mathias, 1977; Delgado, 1996a; Fisch, 1968; Spencer-Molloy, 1994) and restaurants (Hernandez, 1994; Raynor, 1991; Stout, 1988) have received superficial attention.

Bodegas and restaurants, like their religious counterparts, provide a variety of social support services that supplement the primary commercial-interests of the establishment (Delgado, 1996b). These establishments provide at least seven key services to the Puerto Rican community in general, and the elder population specifically: (1) counseling (Agins, 1985: Vazquez, 1975); (2) cultural connectedness to homeland (Rohter, 1985a; Raynor, 1991; Rierden, 1992; Vazquez, 1974); (3) assistance in filling out or interpreting government forms (Howe, 1984; Vazquez, 1974); (4) community-related news and information (Agins, 1985; Korrol, 1983; Terry, 1992); (5) information and referral to social service agencies (Howe, 1986; Vazquez, 1974); (6) credit (Agins, 1985; Fitzpatrick, 1987); and (7) banking–check cashing (Fitzpartick, 1987; Howe, 1986).

However, there are many other types of merchant establishments in the Puerto Rican community that are highly visible and accessible to elders and other age groups (Rohter, 1985b, c; Stout, 1988). The paucity of information on these institutions raises important questions for the field of gerontology: (1) Are these institutions providing social services and leadership in helping Puerto Rican elder customers? (2) Are the support roles similar or different from those reported in the literature for food and religious establishments? (3) What services, if any, can be considered unique to these establishments? Answers to these questions are very important in the development of a more comprehensive picture of Puerto Rican elder natural caregiving systems, a picture that undoubtedly highlights both the richness and complexity of these systems.

DESCRIPTION OF SETTING AND STUDY

This article is based upon data gathered in Holyoke, Massachusetts (Delgado, 1995c). Holyoke is located in the western part of the state, approximately 100 miles west of Boston and 60 miles north of Hartford, Connecticut. The city of Holyoke has an overall population of 44,000, of which approximately 28.9 percent are Puerto Rican (12,700); Puerto Ricans are the largest Latino sub-group representing 93.5 percent of all Latinos (Gaston, 1992).

The Puerto Rican community is also the fastest growing population group in Holyoke, with an increase in representation from 5,760 in 1980 to 12,700 in 1990–a 120 percent increase in ten years (Gaston, 1992, 1994). The Puerto Rican elder (over 65 years of age) population more than doubled (114.8 percent) over a ten year period from 142 in 1980 to 305 in 1990 (Gaston Institute, 1992). In 1990 their poverty rate was 35.1 percent (65 to 74 years of age) and 27.3 percent (75 years of age and over) respectively, the highest of any ethnic group in Holyoke (Gaston Institute, 1994).

The data reported in this article were part of a broader study that gathered asset data on religious (Pentecostal) and merchant establishments (food and non-food related institutions). Data were gathered on a forty-block section of Holyoke (commercial and residential section). There were two distinct research phases: (1) the initial phase consisted of interviewers identifying all Puerto Rican/Latino establishments within the study area and gathering key identifying information; and (2) the second phase entailed an in-depth interview with the owner of the establishment; this interview was conducted in Spanish and lasted approximately thirty minutes. Interviewers would meet at the end of the work day and participate in a "debriefing" session during which they would share experiences, reactions, etc.

Food establishments covered grocery stores and restaurants; non-food merchant establishments covered six types found in the community (clothing, gift, and furniture stores, beauty parlors, botanical shops and radio stations). A total of thirteen commercial establishments were interviewed during the winter of 1993-1994; of this total one establishment refused to complete the interview and provided minimal information on their business.

FINDINGS

Social service organizations need to become more cognizant of the operational characteristics of merchant establishments in order to meaningfully engage them in collaborative activities (Delgado, 1996b); in addition, agencies need to have a better understanding of the types of services provided by merchant institutions. Familiarity with operational and service provision will enhance the likelihood of collaborative efforts succeeding in reaching out to the community (Delgado, 1995).

Data were gathered on four operational dimensions: (1) years in operation; (2) hours open; (3) number of days opened per week; and (4) days of the week in operation. This information, in turn, can assist agencies in approaching merchant establishments and in the planning of activities for elders.

The typical establishment had been opened three years. As noted in Table 1, almost half of the establishments (5 out of 12) had been opened one year or less ("B," "C," "D," "F," and "M"). Three-quarters (8 out of 12) had been opened under four years; in essence, these establishments, with one exception ("H"), were relatively new to the community.

The typical establishment is open six days per week–only two were open seven days ("K" and "M"), one was open five days ("F"). Merchant establishments operated an average of 9.4 hours per day with a range of eight hours ("B" and "D") to twenty-four hours ("M")–the latter was a radio station. Most of the merchant establishments were opened Monday through Saturday, 9 A.M. to 6 P.M.

In turning to provision of social services, there is no doubt that merchant establishments, like their religious and food establishment counterparts, are fulfilling multiple roles within the Puerto Rican community. The services they provide, however, are limited to just a few types.

As noted in Table 2, the average merchant establishment provided 2.83 types of services, from a low of two ("E," "H," "K," and "M") to a high of four ("D" and "F"), considerably lower than religious and food establishments. Three services (integration of the lonely, interpreter services, and community leadership) were cited by at least three-fourths of the establish-

TABLE 1. Summary of Descriptive Data

INST.	YEARS OF OPERATION NUMBER OF HOURS OPEN	DAYS OF THE WEEK OPEN							TOTAL NUMBER OF DAYS OPEN
		MON	TUE	WED	THU	FRI	SAT	SUN	
A	3 YEARS 10 HOURS	X	X	X	X	X	X		6
B	5 MONTHS 8 HOURS	X	X	X	X	X	X		6
C	1 YEAR 9 HOURS	X	X	X	X	X	X		6
D	2 MONTHS 8 HOURS	X	X	X	X	X	X		6
E	4 YEARS 7 HOURS	X	X	X	X	X	X		6
F	3 MONTHS 9 HOURS		X	X	X	X	X		5
G	3 YEARS 9 1/2 HOURS	X	X	X	X	X	X		6
H	15 YEARS 10 HOURS	X	X	X	X	X	X		6
I	NO RESPONSE								
J	2 1/2 YEARS 10 HOURS	X	X	X	X	X	X		6
K	5 YEARS 9 HOURS	X	X	X	X	X	X	X	7
L	2 YEARS 8 HOURS	X	X	X	X	X	X		6
M	2 MONTHS 24 HOURS	X	X	X	X	X	X	X	7
		11	12	12	12	12	12	2	X = 6.08

TABLE 2. Summary of Service Provision

TYPE OF SERVICE (Merchant Establishments*)	A	B	C	D	E	F	G	H	I	J	K	L	M	NUMBER OF INST. OFFERING SERVICE
1. Credit														0
2. Information/ Referral													X	1
3. Lonely Integ.	X	X	X	X	X	X	X	X		X	X	X		11
4. Interpreter Services	X	X	X	X	X	X	X	X		X		X		10
5. Counseling														0
6. Donations (Money/Food)				X		X								2
7. Leadership	X	X	X	X		X	X			X		X	X	9
8. Childcare											X			1
NUMBER OF SERVICES PER INSTITUTION	3	3	3	4	2	4	3	2	NO ANS.	3	2	3	2	X = 2.83

* A total of 13 merchant establishments were involved in this study; each establishment is represented with a letter of the alphabet.

39

ments. The first two have great significance for elders. These services, incidently, were also found to be frequently provided by religious and food establishments.

Integration of the lonely (N = 11), the most frequently cited service, generally consisted of providing opportunities for community residents, particularly elders, to interact/connect with merchant personnel and other residents; these merchant settings facilitated Puerto Ricans meeting and socially interacting.

Provision of interpreter services was cited by ten establishments. This service consisted of any or all of the following activities: (1) assistance in reading and interpreting "official" government correspondence for those with limited or no English reading abilities; (2) assistance in filling out government related forms; and (3) telephone calls to government agencies and act as interpreters/advocates for customers (Delgado, 1996b). One institution noted that Puerto Rican elders were the group that most needed this service since many either did not know how to read in English or Spanish. Several government/social agencies did mail elders letters in Spanish. However, elders were either reluctant (pride) orhad great difficulty in conveying to these institutions that they were illiterate in both languages.

Community leadership, the third most frequently cited service (N = 9), consisted of any or all of the following activities: "(1) sponsoring of community events and festivals; (2) donations to other organizations that provide social services (money, supplies, services); (3) allowing community to use space to conduct meetings; (4) membership on agency boards and advisory committees; and (5) allowing community organizations to place posters or distribute information on services" (Delgado, 1996b).

The remaining five services the questionnaire sought information on played minimal or no support roles within the establishments. Only two institutions ("D" and "F") donated services or money to the "poor"; one ("K") provided emergency child care and one ("M") provided elders with information/referrals to social service agencies. Two services usually associated with Puerto Rican establishments (provision of credit and counseling) were not mentioned by any merchant institution.

IMPLICATIONS FOR COLLABORATION

The nature and extent of caregiving support provided by Puerto Rican merchant establishments was not extensive–an average of 2.83 services (5 different types of services). Merchant establishments, in comparison with religious (Pentecostal) and food (grocery store and restaurants) establishments in the same geographical area, are playing a less significant support role. Pentecostal churches provided an average of 7.3 services (16 different types) and food establishments provided an average of 3.36 services (7 different types). However, this should not come as a surprise in light of the high representation of elders in Pentecostal churches and the prominent role of religion in their lives (Carraballo, 1990; Delgado, 1996a).

The lesser caregiving role for merchant establishments may be the result of an interplay of several factors: (1) the relatively recent establishment of these businesses–merchant institutions had been in existence an average of 3.65 years (Pentecostal churches had been opened an average of 6.0 years and food establishments an average of 4.6 years); (2) the lack of counseling and information referral services (only one institution noted information-referral) may be due to a lack of familiarity with, or lack of outreach by, social agencies; (3) customers may not expect merchant institutions to play active caregiving roles; and (4) the nature of the service/product that is sold does not lend itself to frequent and sustained contact with customers–thus, merchant establishments are not frequented as often as food establishments or religious institutions.

Nevertheless, the limited role that merchant establishments play in the community highlights a potential for more active involvement in assisting elders, if provided with an opportunity and appropriate resources. It is important to keep in mind that virtually all of these institutions provided a setting for the lonely to connect, served as interpreters for customers, and were involved in various community-wide events/activities.

Social agencies wishing to collaborate with merchant institutions must first be prepared to spend a period of time becoming familiar with these establishments (Delgado, 1996a). It is essential that personal contact transpire to be better aware of the types of people they serve, how business is conducted, what kind of services they provide that are supportive in nature, etc., (Delgado, 1995). In essence, it is necessary to enter a phase that can best be described as relationship building. This phase will provide social service agencies with invaluable information concerning which establishments are interested in a collaborative relationship and which have a high number of elder customers; not all merchant establishments may be interested (Delgado, 1994).

An information-sharing phase will follow during which social agencies can enlist the support of merchants in disseminating information on elder services or posting of notices. For some establishments this may very well be the extent of collaboration. However, there may be institutions that wish to establish referral procedures and utilize agency contact persons to make referrals. This service delivery phase offers tremendous promise. Merchant establishments, for example, may provide space for community workshops–these institutions may be large enough to have space for group meetings; these establishments, it must be remembered, offer the advantages of being located within the community and are, as already noted, accessible geographically, psychologically, logistically, and culturally.

This collaborative phase may also entail an exchange of resources–merchant establishments may sponsor community activities, donate money, merchandise, and services to agencies; social agencies, in turn, may purchase services, materials, or, rent space, to list just three possibilities. In short, both sectors (formal and natural) can enter into formalized/non-formalized contractual agreements (Delgado, 1995b).

The community leadership role played by merchant establishments provides an excellent avenue for enlisting potential elder board/advisory committee members. It is important to note that including community representatives on agency committees increases the likelihood of services being culture-specific (Delgado, under review). Merchants are also in key positions to have a sense of community assets and needs and should be included in any assessment of a community, i.e., key informant surveys.

The potential for increasing community involvement in all phases of service delivery is greatly enhanced when social service organizations are prepared to enter into a meaningful and co-equal collaborative process. This process entails learning about the other party, sharing information, and entering into a partnership where all sides benefit. This is particularly critical in reaching out to elders who may be isolated and in great need.

CONCLUSION

A shift in paradigms from viewing communities as problem-ridden to possessing strengths/resources, necessitates an expansive view of community. This article has focused on an often overlooked natural caregiving system in the lives of Puerto Rican elders; merchant institutions are highly visible and fulfill important support roles. However, the professional literature, and possibly practitioners/social agencies, have largely ignored this resource.

It is important to understand that not all merchant establishments may be interested in collaboration, just like not all agencies may be interested in this type of relationship (Delgado, 1995c). It becomes particularly critical that an assessment be made to ascertain the willingness and ability of merchant institutions to engage in collaboration. This assessment process cannot be accomplished without bilingual, and preferably, bi-cultural staff, who are very knowledgeable of the Puerto Rican elders and the community in general. Collaboration with a merchant establishment that has a reputation for unethical practices will be detrimental to an agency; conversely, collaborating with a merchant institution that has an impeccable reputation, can prove extremely beneficial.

The field of gerontology is in an excellent position to "re-discover" communities and develop innovative ways for identifying and developing community resources (Delgado, 1996c). The use of merchant establishments in Puerto Rican communities across the United States is one such approach; other undervalued communities in the United States, too, have resources that must be acknowledged and utilized to the betterment of communities in general, and elders in particular.

REFERENCES

Agins, T. (March 15, 1985). To Hispanics in U.S., a bodega, or grocery, is a vital part of life. *The Wall Street Journal*, 1, 6, 13.

Barrera, Jr., M. & Reese, F. (1993). Natural support systems and Hispanic substance abuse. In R.S. Mayers, B.L. Kail & T.D. Watts (Eds.), *Hispanic substance abuse* (pp. 115-130). Springfield, IL: Charles C Thomas Publishers.

Borrello, M.A. and Mathias, E. (1977). Botanicas: Puerto Rican folk pharmacies. *Natural History*, 86, 64-73.

Boston Persistent Poverty Project. (1989). *In the midst of plenty: A profile of Boston and its poor.* Boston, MA: The Boston Foundation.

Burros, M. (July 18, 1990). Supermarkets reach out to Hispanic customers. *The New York Times*, C1, C6.

Caraballo, E.R. (1990). *The role of the Pentecostal church as a service provider in the Puerto Rican community in Boston, Massachusetts: A case study.* Waltham, MA: Doctoral Dissertation, Brandeis University.

Carmody, D. (May 2, 1972). Bodega owners gain strength in co-op here. *The New York Times*, 31.

Carr, E. and Perez, A. (May 16, 1993). The rites of the ancient ones: Spiritualists are often regarded as charlatans, but to practioners a visit to a curandero is as spiritual as a Sunday church service. *Los Angeles Times*, 16.

Carrasquillo, H. (1994). The Puerto Rican family. In R.L. Taylor (Ed.), *Minority families in the United States: A multicultural perspective* (pp. 82-94). Englewood Cliffs, NJ: Prentice Hall Publishing Co.

Daley, J. M. & Wong, P. (1994). Community development with emerging ethnic communities. *Journal of Community Practice*, 1, 9-24.

Deck, A. F. and Nunez, J.A. (October 23,1982). Religious enthusiasm and Hispanic youth. *America*, 232-234.

De La Rosa, M. (1988). Natural support systems of Hispanic Americans: A key dimension of wellbeing. *Health and Social Work*, 13, 181-190.

Delgado, M. (1996a). Puerto Rican elders and botanical shops: A community resource or liability? *Social Work in Health Care*, 23, 67-81.

Delgado, M. (1996b). Puerto Rican food establishments as social service organizations: Results of an asset assessment. *Journal of Community Practice*, 3, 57-77.

Delgado, M. (1996c). Aging research and the Puerto Rican community: The use of an advisory committee of intended respondents. *The Gerontologist*, 36, 406-408.

Delgado, M. (1995a). Puerto Rican elders and natural support systems: Implications for human services. *Journal of Gerontological Social Work*, 24, 115-130.

Delgado, M. (1995b). Hispanic natural support systems and alcohol and other drug services: Challenges and rewards for practice. *Alcoholism Treatment Quarterly,* 12 (1), 17-31.

Delgado, M. (1995c). Community asset assessment and substance abuse prevention: A case study involving the Puerto Rican community. *Journal of Child & Adolescent Substance Abuse,* 4, 57-77.

Delgado, M. (1994). Hispanic natural support systems and the alcohol and drug abuse field: A developmental framework for collaboration. *Journal of Multi-Cultural Social Work,* 3, 11-37.

Delgado, M. & Humm-Delgado, D. (1982). Natural support systems: Source of strength in Hispanic communities. *Social Work,* 1982, 27, 83-89.

Delgado, M. & Rosati, M. (Pending publication). Religion, asset assessment and AOD: A case study of a Puerto Rican community in Massachusetts. *Journal of Health & Social Policy.*

Eckenrode, J. (Ed.). (1991). *The social context of coping.* New York: Plenum Press.

Fisch, S. (1968). Botanicas and spiritism in a metropolis. *Milbank Memorial Fund,* 41, 377-388.

Fitzpatrick, J.P. (1987). *Puerto Rican Americans: The meaning of migration to the mainland.* Englewood Cliffs, NJ: Prentice Hall Publishers.

Gaiter, D.J. (December 24, 1980). At Christmas, Hispanic Pentecostal church puts stress on 'gifts' without price tags. *The New York Times,* B1, B4.

Garrido, M. (1988). *Human services needs and help-seeking patterns in a community of Puerto Ricans in New Jersey.* New Brunswick, NJ: Dissertation, Graduate School of Applied and Professional Psychology, Rutgers University.

Gaston Institute. (1992). *Latinos in Holyoke.* Boston, MA: University of Massachusetts.

Gaston Institute. (1994). *Latinos in Holyoke: poverty, income, education, employment, and housing.* Boston, MA: University of Massachusetts.

Ghali, S.B. (1982). Understanding Puerto Rican traditions. *Social Work,* 27, 98-102.

Glugoski, G., Reisch, M. and Rivera, F.G. (1994). A wholistic ethno-cultural paradigm: A new model for community organization teaching and practice. *Journal of Community Practice,* 1, 81-98.

Gonzales, D. (September 1, 1992) Dominican immigration alters Hispanic New York. *The New York Times,* Section A, 1.

Gutierrez, L.M. and Ortega, R.M. (1991). Developing methods to empower Latinos: The importance of groups. *Social Work With Groups,* 14, 23-43.

Gutierrez, L., Ortega, R.M., Suarez, Z. (1990). Self-help and the Latino community: In T.J. Powell (Ed.), *Working with self-help* (pp. 218-236). Silver Springs, MD: National Association of Social Workers.

Harwood, A. (1977). *Rx: Spiritist as needed: A study of a Puerto Rican community mental health resource.* New York: John Wiley & Sons.

Hernandez, R. (July 12, 1994). Where Hispanic merchants thrive: In Westchester, growth of businesses bolsters economy. *The New York Times,* 1.

Howe, M. (November 19, 1986). Bodegas find prosperity amid change. *The New York Times,* 8.

Korrol, V.E.S. (1983). *From colonia to community: The history of Puerto Ricans in New York City, 1917-1948.* Westport, CT: Greenwood Press.

Kretzmann, J.P. and McKnight, J.L. (1993). *Building communities from the inside out: A path toward finding and mobilizing a community's assets.* Evanston, IL: Center for Urban Affairs and Policy Research, Northwestern University.

Longres, J.F. (1988). *Human behavior in the social environment.* Itasca, IL: F.E. Peacock Publishers, Inc.

Martin, J.M. and Martin, E.P. (1985). *The helping tradition in the Black family and community.* Washington, D.C.: National Association of Social Workers.

Mason, J.L. (1994). Developing culturally competent organizations. *Focal Point, 8,* 1-8.

Morales, J. (1992). Community social work in Puerto Rican communities in the United States: One organizer's perspective. In F. Rivera & J. Ehrlich (Eds.), *Community organization in a diverse society* (pp. 110-118). Boston, MA: Allyn & Bacon Publishers.

Raynor, V. (July 7, 1991). Charting the migration of Puerto Ricans, and their resilience. *The New York Times,* 14.

Rierden, A. (February 16, 1992). Problems temper Puerto Ricans' success. *The New York Times,* Section 12 CN, 1.

Rivera, Jr., G. (1990). AIDS and Mexican folk medicine. *Social Science Research,* 75, 3-7.

Rogler, L.H. and Cooney, R.S. (1984). *Puerto Rican families in New York City: Intergenerational processes.* Maplewood, NJ: Waterfront Press.

Rohter, L. (Saturday, January 12, 1985a). Protestantism gaining influence in Hispanic community. *The New York Times,* 23, 26.

Rohter, L. (August 11, 1985b). New York's thriving Hispanic banks. *The New York Times,* 4.

Rohter, L. (October 10, 1985c). El Barrio residents worry and wait. *The New York Times,* Section B, 16.

Sanchez, C. (1987). Self-help: Model for strengthening the informal support system of the Hispanic elderly. *Journal of Gerontological Social Work,* 9, 117-130.

Sanchez-Ayendez, M. (1988). Puerto Rican elderly women: The cultural dimension of social support network. *Women & Health,* 14, 239-252.

Spencer-Molloy, F. (March 2, 1994). Doctor negotiates path between folk and traditional medicines. *The Hartford Courant,* D9.

Stout, H. (June 26, 1988). What's new in Hispanic business: Out of the Barrio and into the mainstream. *The New York Times,* 13.

Terry, S. (August 22, 1992). A wave of immigration is fast changing Boston. *The New York Times,* 5.

Thompson, M.S. & Peebles-Wilkins, W. (1992) The impact of formal, informal, and societal support networks on the psychological well-being of Black adolescent mothers. *Social Work,* 37, 322-328.

Vazquez, J.D. (1974). La Bodega–A social institution. *In the Puerto Rican curriculum development workshop: A report,* (pp. 31-36). New York: Council on Social Work Education.

Williams, S.E. & Wright, D.F. (1992). Empowerment: The strengths of Black families revisited. *Journal of Multi-Cultural Social Work,* 2, 23-36.

The Yaqui Elderly of Old Pascua

Juan Paz, DSW
Sara Aleman, PhD

BACKGROUND

This paper is an exploratory study using survey research methods to explore the social and economic well being and health status of the Yaqui elderly in Old Pascua Village in Tucson, Arizona. The main theory tested in this study is that poverty and oppression are two overarching variables affecting the health care of Yaqui elders. Presently there is a paucity of literature and research on the health care status of the Yaqui elderly. These research findings are further utilized culturally competent for social work practice. In consideration of the Yaqui culture's enmeshment with the Mexican American and other indigenous cultures, the researchers have utilized available literature of these other groups. The Yaqui lifestyle and culture shares much in common with these groups.

The Yaqui people are an indigenous population with origins in the Mexican state of Sonora adjacent to Arizona. The Yaqui are known as "indios" in the Rio Yaqui Pacific Coast region of Sonora, Mexico. In the United States they are referred to as Native American. The experience of the Yaqui elderly has been one where they have been historically excluded from participating fully in social services programs. They often encountered barriers to needed social services. This has contributed to conditions of chronic poverty among the elderly.

Juan Paz is affiliated with Arizona State University. Sara Aleman is affiliated with Northern Arizona University.

[Haworth co-indexing entry note]: "The Yaqui Elderly of Old Pascua." Paz, Juan, and Sara Aleman. Co-published simultaneously in *Journal of Gerontological Social Work* (The Haworth Press, Inc.) Vol. 30, No. 1/2, 1998, pp. 47-59; and: *Latino Elders and the Twenty-First Century: Issues and Challenges for Culturally Competent Research and Practice* (ed: Melvin Delgado) The Haworth Press, Inc., 1998, pp. 47-59. Single or multiple copies of this article are available for a fee from The Haworth Document Delivery Service [1-800-342-9678, 9:00 a.m. - 5:00 p.m. (EST). E-mail address: getinfo@haworthpressinc.com].

47

RATIONALE

Using quantitative measures from the OARS questionnaire, the well being of the elderly was studied using the variables of annual income, sources of income, family income and living arrangements. Barriers to social services such as transportation and language were also studied. A qualitative/ historical approach was used to study the historical oppression that Yaqui elderly have experienced in order to understand their current reality.

METHODOLOGY

The OARS questionnaire originally used to assess the health status of senior citizens in the United States (Pfeiffer, 1976) was selected to assess the health status of the Yaqui elderly. A Spanish language version of the questionnaire previously used to study the Cuban elderly in Miami, Florida was modified (Santisteban & Szapocznik, 1981) to reflect the Spanish being used in Old Pascua. Two Yaqui key informants were used to review the protocol for its cultural and language appropriateness. The questionnaire underwent a process of translation from English to Spanish and then from Spanish to English in order to safeguard that the meaning of the questions not be changed in the translation process (Santisteban & Szapocznik, 1981).

During the spring of 1995, students in a graduate social work class designed to teach minority content conducted the interviews of the entire sample. Students received 20 hours of training on interviewing skills. Research teams of two would conduct the interviews at either the senior citizens center or their homes. All of the research teams had one Spanish speaking person who would conduct the interview. The other student would record the interview.

SAMPLE

The study was composed of a purposive sample. A total of 85 persons were interviewed which comprises almost all of the elderly in the community except for a few homebound elderly. The Old Pascua community is small in size numbering approximately 722 persons. A total of 469 enrolled Yaqui live in the Old Pascua Village It was decided to collect the data at the tribe's senior citizens center where the majority of the elderly participate in daily nutrition and social activities. It is the researchers' perspective that the data collected reflects the reality of the Old Pascua elderly.

Members of the Pascua Yaqui Tribe state-wide now number 10,000. This figure includes enrolled Yaqui and Yaqui who are pending enrollment. This does not include the number of descendants who are not registered with the tribe. There are 7,180 registered tribal members who live in six traditional Yaqui communities in Arizona (U.S. Department of Commerce, 1992). Old Pascua Village, the oldest of the Tucson Yaqui barrios, is located in central Tucson. Before analysis of the research findings, it is necessary to understand the historical context of the Yaqui elderly and how it has contributed to the current well being.

Historical Survival and Oppression

During the end of the 1800s and the early part of this century, the Yaqui migrated to the United States because in the Rio Yaqui area they were being persecuted and killed by the Mexican government. The dictator Porfirio Diaz implemented a policy that resulted in the extermination of thousands of Yaqui, much in the same manner that Jewish people were exterminated during World War II.

According to Turner, in his historical accounts of Mexico, 15,700 Yaquis were sold into slavery to work in Yucatan in the henequen plantations during 1905 alone. They were sold at the price of 65 pesos each (Turner, 1985). Two-thirds died within the first year of slavery. Diaz' goal was to "appropriate the rich lands of the Yaqui nation and quell their constant rebellions against the national government, thousands were deported to the henequen plantation of Yucatan, while some were sent to Tuxtepec, Tabasco, and Chiapas" (Chassen-Lopez, 1997). Some Yaqui individuals left their villages and went to live in the larger towns, learning the Spanish language and Mexican culture to avoid persecution. Some intermarried with Mexicans while others migrated to the United States and founded several communities in Arizona. In Tucson, people first moved into Old Pascua Village at the turn of the 20th century; it was officially founded in 1921.

In Arizona, the Yaqui experience is one of marginalization and historical oppression. Like other tribes in the United States, they have also experienced inequities and barriers to social services (U.S. Commission on Civil Rights, 1982). Similarly, they have also experienced the injustices faced by Mexican American groups along the Southwest border area.

In 1952, Pascua Village was annexed into the City of Tucson, where the Yaqui still live. They waged a long and difficult battle to secure federal recognition. On September 18, 1978, Public Law 95-375 was signed into law granting the Pascua Yaqui of Arizona the same status as all other federally recognized Native American tribes in the United States (Spicer, 1984; 1985).

The Current Cohort of the Yaqui Elderly

The Yaqui elderly population of Old Pascua comprises a generation of Yaqui who are children of the first generation who migrated to Old Pascua

Village in Tucson from their coastal villages in Sonora, Mexico. This cohort of elderly has been marginalized since childhood. Their parents often came to this country seeking safety from persecution by the Mexican government. Life within Old Pascua Village provided safety from persecution for their families. Their families developed strong patterns of self reliance. Individuals in need sought help from within the community to avoid government intervention (Holden, 1991). However, it was understood by the community members that the poor, "los pobres," are individuals who have exhausted all their resources and are in need of basic assistance, "tienen necesidad."

Social service agencies for the most part have been located outside the Yaqui community, making transportation and access to services a significant barrier. In 1982, the United States Commission on Civil Rights noted the existence of barriers to senior citizens programs in Tucson. Participation by Hispanics and Native Americans was minimal in relation to their representation in Pima County's population. In 1988 a senior citizens center was created within Old Pascua Village adjacent to the Neighborhood Youth Center.

The Yaqui culture is one that recognizes the worth and dignity of all individuals. The elderly are well respected and play a significant and powerful role in their society. This is the opposite from the current political ethos. Agency social workers under the current mandate to serve the "worthy poor" often treat Yaqui elders with disrespect and without concern for their dignity. Agency representatives are more concerned with the large amount of red tape (Yeatts, Crow & Folts, 1992).

RESULTS

Demographics

The reality of the Yaqui elderly is one of pervasive poverty. Examination of the variables related to income indicates patterns of chronic poverty which reflect the reality of the current cohort of Yaqui elderly. They have spent a lifetime working in labor and agriculture, both low paying occupations.

The sample population included 36 males and 49 females. Table 1 illustrates some similarities between the Yaqui elderly and the Mexican American elderly. The Yaqui elderly are beginning to identify as older persons at a younger age because they are experiencing the problems of aging earlier than other groups. Nearly one-third, 28.9% were are from ages 55-64. Nearly half, 47% are from age 65 to 74. These are the young-old. From the remainder, 13.3% were from age 75-84, while 2.4% were from age 85-91. Clearly the majority of the elderly are at the young-old age spectrum.

The vast majority (93%) identified as either Hispanic or Yaqui and speak

TABLE 1. Age by Gender of Yaqui Elders

Age Values	Males (N)	Females (N)	Valid percent
45-54	4	3	8.4
55-64	7	17	28.9
65-74	15	24	47.0
75-84	6	5	13.3
85-91	2	0	2.4
Totals	34	49	100.0

Number of missing observations: 2

Spanish only; a smaller number speak Cahiti which is the Yoeme language. This dual identity is understandable because in the past some elderly identified themselves and their families as Mexican American for survival and safety. Still others identified as Native American because they shared similar experiences with the Tohono O'Odham. The Tohono O'Odham, like the Yaqui, have their roots in Mexico and are a binational, trilingual group. Consequently, they also share a strong bond with Mexico.

The majority of the elderly (60%) have six or less years of education and only 8 persons had more than a high school education. Close to half (49%) of the sample were married while 11 were single. An additional 4 persons were separated, 5 were divorced, and 23 were widowed.

Income

Approximately one-third of the sample have retired. In addition, one-quarter of the sample was retired on disability; only 12 of the respondents had income from earnings. A significantly large number of individuals (74%) are dependent on social security benefits for their incomes. An even larger number (80%) make an annual income of less than $7,000 per year. Table 2 provides a breakdown of income by age. The data in this table strengthens the notion that a significant number live in poverty with few sources of income. In addition, one-fifth (21%) are receiving Supplemental SSI Benefits. From the remainder, 15% receive money from a retirement pension.

Intergenerational Families and Poverty

A significantly large portion of the population live in Intergenerational families. These are defined as households where several generations of the

TABLE 2. Income by Age of Yaqui Elders

Income	45-54	55-64	65-74	75-84	85+
0-$2999	2	7	2	3	0
$3000-$6000	4	8	25	6	2
$7000-$9999	1	4	8	1	0
$10000+	0	4	3	0	0
Total	7 (8.8%)	23 (28.8%)	38 (47.5%)	10 (12.5%)	2 (2.5%)

family live together. Nearly half (48%) reported living with their children, slightly over one-quarter (28%) have grandchildren who live with them, and approximately one-tenth (11%) have other relatives living with them. The data reveal that almost half (44%) of the respondents live in households with three members or more. This compares to a majority elderly population that has an average of 2.5 family household members (Jimenez & Figueiredo, 1994; John, 1995).

In spite of these predominant intergenerational living arrangements, the household income level is consistently low. The majority of elders reported they live with family members. Only one person reported receiving financial assistance from their family on a regular basis. This striking fact is indicative of two important pieces of information. One, is that in most Yaqui families, the elderly are a major source of economic support for the family system. Second, is that most intergenerational families live in poverty. The second fact is consistent with other Native American and Mexican family experiences. Overall, these data suggest that a large number of Yaqui households survive in conditions of poverty. Income data from the study reveal that, in one-third of the households, two persons live on one income. Close to half (48%) of households have three or more persons dependent on one person's income.

Further analysis of living arrangements revealed that 47.6% of respondents live in husband/wife primary households. This number compares to 49% of Hispanic elders who live with a spouse (Commonwealth Commission Fund, 1989). These groups reflect higher rates of spousal relationships in later years than does the majority elderly population as reflected in the OARS results (Pfeiffer, 1976).

In the exploration of factors that may contribute to poverty, the related issues of receipt of social security and marital status cannot be disregarded

(Popple & Leighninger, 1996). Some researchers (Atchely, 1991; Hopper, 1993) have found that being married is an important factor in staying out of poverty; others have found that elders who live alone are most likely to live in chronic poverty. This is consistent with studies that show that American Indians and Hispanics in single headed households are more likely to be in poverty (Arizona Community Association, Inc., 1994; U.S. Department of Health and Human Services, 1987).

These data demonstrate that the elderly and their families possess limited economic resources and live in Intergenerational families to cope with the hardships of chronic poverty. The variables of income and living arrangements must not be confused with housing preference. Some Hispanic researchers state that the elderly have a preference for intergenerational living. Not so; "la necesidad," the need to live with a minimally decent quality of life, often forces them to live in Intergenerational households (Paz, 1986). In fact, an earlier study conducted by Glugoski (personal communication, 1995) of Hispanic elderly in California found that if given the option and if it were economically feasible a majority of the elderly would elect to live in their own homes.

Triple Jeopardy

These data strengthen the theory that Yaqui elders experience triple jeopardy, (i.e., old, poor and members of an ethnic minority group). They face social and historical barriers that prevent their participation in programs designed for senior citizens. This cohort of elderly live in an urban setting. In some cases they are excluded from receiving health care and social services because they do not live on a reservation. Historically, issues of language, transportation and mistrust of government prevent their access to needed services. For example, during the 1980s the umbrella agency, the Pima Council on Aging and Tucson Metropolitan Ministries, operated a meals program for Yaqui elders. Participants in the meals program were first obliged to accept a diet of foods designed for white senior citizens. Nine years ago, the tribe took over the nutrition program and hired Yaqui individuals to prepare nutritional meals that incorporated their dietary preferences.

The Yaqui elderly find themselves in a state of social services limbo where they are often denied services and forced to go without them. Originally they were denied services because they were thought to be Mexican nationals making them ineligible for state services. On the other hand, some health care planners categorized them as being Native American making them ineligible to receive health care services. For example, the state managed health care system for the poor, known as the Arizona Health Care Cost Containment System, often excluded Yaqui elders from receiving services. These individuals were compelled to apply for services financed by the Indian Health Services (IHS). Nevertheless, when these senior citizens sought services financed by IHS, they were denied services because they were not enrolled Native Americans. When older individuals received services from a community health center, they encountered several days of waiting for an appointment and frequently were met with a dehumanizing amount of bureaucratic red tape. Some individuals went without services due to negative experiences with the system. Avoidance of the health and social service network is often seen as a way to preserve their dignity.

Transportation Services

Transportation is a major barrier to the Yaqui because the Old Pascua Yaqui community is located a significant distance from most health care and social services. Access to services is a major issue for the elderly. Over half (61%) are provided transportation to and from services by a member of their family. Slightly over one-fifth (22.4%) rely on public transportation to get to the services they need. Only 11 persons or 12.9% of the sample reported they receive transportation services from a public agency. Subsequently, when asked whether or not they were satisfied with the transportation services they received, only 25.9% answered in the affirmative.

Language Discrimination

As mentioned earlier, Spanish is the language of choice for the majority of the elderly. Some do speak Cahiti and English. When the data collection process was underway for this project, some discussion was held with the elderly about their experiences with agencies serving senior citizens. The majority of the elderly indicated that many agencies still do not have bilingual workers and that still other agencies required them to take their own translator along. This often discouraged them from seeking services, since getting to the agency alone was a challenge.

Adequate Income and Expenses

The expenditures of these elders suggest dire financial straits when we see the data on income. Among those that pay rent, 9% pay $50 to $99, 26% pay $100 to $149, 26% pay $150 to $199, and 26% pay from $200 to $349. While this rent may seem small in comparison to other urban areas, the amount is significantly more than 25% of income when utilities and maintenance costs are added. Food is another area of financial concern. The majority (80%) pay for all of their own food. Only a small percentage (9.4%) receive food stamps benefits. In fact when asked if they needed food stamps 46% answered in the affirmative. The study's participants were also asked whether they had sufficient finances to meet emergencies. The vast majority (72%) indicated they did not. When further queried whether or not they needed financial help again, 72% indicated they did.

IMPLICATIONS FOR SOCIAL WORK PRACTICE

Social work practice with Yaqui elderly clients requires practitioners to have a planning stage. In the planning stage the social worker would work with the client to prepare for interaction with a health care and social services network that is often hostile to persons from diverse cultural backgrounds (Chestang, 1972). In other words, they need to prepare the client to deal with agencies that do not value diversity. If this preparation is not done, the distrust of the Yaqui elderly client can easily be heightened by exposure to an agency that is culturally insensitive. For example, an agency may require a person to bring their own translator to an interview or may not provide any privacy to discuss personal problems.

The planning stage, for example, may include preparing a client for rejection from eligibility for services as well as the aforementioned intrusions into private matters. In cases where services are denied, clients need to be informed of options such as filing an appeal, challenging a decision and/or involving the assistance of a legal aid center or other possible advocates. Preparing a client for possible rejection from services is vital especially in cases where persons have never asked for assistance. Rejection from services may have serious social and psychological effects on clients by making them feel increasingly vulnerable. The trauma of rejection is compounded by their lose of dignity and respect. The planning stage helps to minimize these problems by acknowledging that eligibility determinations are not always final, may be in error and can be challenged.

Social workers who provide services to Yaqui elders must take into account several variables. The first major variable to consider during the initial stage of conducting an assessment is to include the total family when planning the delivery of services. Instead of viewing the elderly as separate from their family, they should be viewed as inextricably intertwined with their family. In other words, instead of providing only person-based services, the focus should be on providing family-based services which take into consideration the family context in which the elderly live.

This research has uncovered Intergenerational poverty among families. Another social work role entails facilitating the ability of the family to ameliorate their economic status by linking them to services. This requires social workers to develop extensive knowledge of elderly and family services available in the community and to function in the role of a broker. This may be necessary in the case of facilitating access to medical care or food stamps. The broker role will also require the social worker to develop an extensive knowledge of programs and policies that are targeted to Native American, Mexican American and other elderly. The broker will have to develop skills at helping their client population negotiate through the myriad of red tape that is required to participate in programs for the elderly. The task of the social worker is to minimize the negative impact of the red tape and to facilitate the flow of information and services in an expeditious manner.

Culturally competent services to Yaqui elderly necessitate a tri-cultural approach to service delivery. This includes determining the acculturation level of the client. Some Yaqui elders may identify more with the Yaqui culture while others may identify more with the Hispanic culture. Still others may identify with other Native American cultures. An added dimension to their cultural identity is how positive they feel about their own culture. Do they have a positive sense of worth? Are they proud or are they embarrassed of their culture? How long has the client been in the United States? What is the primary language dominance of the client? Some individuals may be Spanish dominant, some may be English dominant and others may be bilingual. Another group may speak the original Yoeme language of their forefathers in addition to their adopted languages. How comfortable is the client dealing with non-Yaqui systems? How comfortable is the client dealing with non-Yaqui persons? Some Yaquis may refuse to seek services outside their community. For example, recently an 80 year old woman was taken to the hospital to receive health care services by a registered nurse. However, the woman's illness was already advanced to the stage where she died within a week. This woman had previously refused to go to a hospital for health care. It was only through the skilled and convincing persuasion of a Yaqui nurse that she finally agreed to go to the hospital. A subsequent discussion with the nurse revealed the elderly woman to be a classic example of an individual who did not trust the health care system and chose to go without needed care.

In recognition of the fact that a high level of distrust exists towards outsiders, social workers must also determine to what extent a client is willing to trust the social worker. From a cultural vantage point, the social worker must begin from the outset to establish bonds of mutual trust, or "confianza," with his client.

In sum, social work practice with poor Yaqui elderly poses a challenge. To be bilingual and bicultural in the Southwest is no longer sufficient. The dynamic interaction of the Yaqui with other populations of the Southwest demonstrates the necessity to be multi-cultural and have the requisite skills to assess the impact of poverty and barriers on the health status and life situation of ethnic elders. Several recommendations arise from this research.

First is the need to have a planning stage during the traditional social work assessment. The purpose is to prepare the client to deal adequately with a potentially hostile system. The second recommendation is to develop a comprehensive approach that identifies resources available in the community and matches them to the client system. The third recommendation is that Yaqui elders must be provided services within the context of their total family system. Social workers must be flexible in instituting action modalities that will require engaging in the broker role on behalf of their clients. And finally, the influence of a client's culture must be considered during all stages of the helping relationship.

REFERENCES

American Society on Aging. (1992). *Serving elders of color: Challenges to providers and the aging network.* Washington, DC: Author.

Arizona Community Action Association, Inc. (1994). *Poverty in Arizona: A Shared Responsibility.* Phoenix, AZ: Author.

Arizona Department of Commerce. (1992, December). *Pascua Yaqui Indian Reservation Community Profile.* Phoenix, AZ: Author.

Atchely, R.C. (1991). *Social forces and aging* (6th ed.). Belmont, CA: Wadsworth Publishing Company.

Chassen-Lopez, F. (1998). In press. *Juana Catarina Romero, Porfirian Cacica: The Woman and the Myth.* University of Kentucky.

Davis, K. (1990). *The Commonwealth Fund Commission on Elderly People Living Alone. National Survey of Hispanic Elderly People, 1988.* [Computer file]. Rockville, MD: Westat, Inc. [producer], 1988. Ann Arbor, MI: Inter-university Consortium for Political and Social Research [distributor].

Devore, W. & Schlesinger, E.G. (1991). *Ethnic-sensitive social work practice* (3rd ed.). New York: Macmillan Publishing Company.

Garcia, A. (1993). Income security and elderly Latinos. In M. Sotomayor & A. Garcia (Eds.), *Elderly Latinos: Issues and solutions for the 21st century* (pp. 2-28). Washington, DC: National Hispanic Council on Aging.

Holden, K.J. (1991). *Yaqui women: Contemporary life histories.* London: University of Nebraska Press.

Holden, W.C., Seltzer, C.C., Studhalter, R.A., Wagner, C.J. & McMillan W.G. (1936). *Studies of the Yaqui Indians of Sonora, Mexico.* Lubbock, TX: Texas Technological College.

Hopper, S.V. (1993). The influence of ethnicity on the health of older women. In F.E. Kaiser (Ed.), *Clinics in geriatric medicine* (pp 231-259). Philadelphia, PA: W.B. Saunders Company.

Jimenez, R.G. & de Figueiredo, J.M. (1994). Issues in the psychiatric care of Hispanic American elders. American Psychiatric Association. (Eds.) *Task Force on Ethnic Minority Elderly,* (pp. 63-90). Washington, DC: American Psychiatric Association.

John, R. (1994). American Indian elders' health, income security, and formal and informal support systems: The need for praxis. In V.G. Griffith (Ed.), *Quarterly*

Journal of the International Institute on Aging. (pp. 1-13). Valleta VLT, Malta: United Nations–Malta.

John, R. (1995). American Indian and Alaska native elders: An assessment of their current status and provision of services. Washington, DC: US Department of Health and Human Services.

Kulys, R. (1990). The ethnic factor in the delivery of social services. In A. Monk (Ed.), *Handbook of gerontological services* (pp. 629-661). New York: Columbia University Press.

Kunitz, S.J., & Levy, J.E. (1991). *Navajo aging.* Tucson, AZ: The University of Arizona Press.

Lacayo, C.G. (1980). *A national study to assess the service needs of the Hispanic elderly: Final report.* Los Angeles, CA: Association Nacional Pro Personas Mayores.

Locust, C. (1987). *Yaqui Indian beliefs about health and handicaps.* Tucson AZ: University of Arizona.

Lopez, C. (1991). *On the sidelines: Hispanic elderly and the continuum of care.* Washington, DC: National Council of La Raza.

Lubben, J.E. & Becerra, R.M. (1987). Social support among Black, Mexican, and Chinese elderly, In D.E. Gelfand & C.M. Barresi (Eds.), *Ethnic dimensions of aging* (pp. 130-140). New York: Springer Publishing Company.

Markides, K.S., & Mindel, C.H. (1987). *Aging and ethnicity.* Newbury Park: Sage Publications.

Paz, J. (1986). "Housing Issues and the Hispanic Elderly." Published by the House Subcommittee on Housing and Community Development. Subcommittee of the House Banking and Commerce Committee. Washington, DC.

Pfeifer, E. (1976). *Multidimensional functional assessment: The OARS methodology.* Durham, NC: Duke University.

Popple, P.R. & Leighninger, L. (1993). *Social work, social welfare, and American society* (2nd ed.). Boston, MA: Allyn & Bacon.

Poverty in Arizona: A People's perspective. (1985). Phoenix, AZ: Arizona Community Action Association, Inc.

Santisteban, D., & Szapocznik, J. 1981. Adaptation of the multidimensional functional assessment questionnaire for use with Hispanic elders.

Schulz, J.H. (1988). *The economics of aging.* Dover, MA: Auburn House Publishing Company.

Spicer, E.H. (1984). *Pascua: A Yaqui Village in Arizona.* Tucson, AZ: The University of Arizona Press.

Spicer, E.H. (1985). *The Yaqui: A cultural history.* Tucson, AZ: The University of Arizona Press.

Turner, J. (1986) *Barbarous Mexico.* Tucson, AZ: University of Arizona Press.

U.S. Commission on Civil Rights. (1982). *Minority elderly services: New programs, old problems, Part I.* Washington, DC: Author.

U.S. Commission on Civil Rights. (1982). *Minority elderly services: New programs old problems, Part II.* Washington, DC: Author

U.S. Department of Commerce. (1992). Pascua Yaqui Indian Reservation Community Profile. Washington, DC.

U.S. Department of Health and Human Services. (1987). *Aging America: Trends and projections*. Washington, DC: Author.

Valle, R. & Martinez, M. (1980). Natural networks of elderly Hispanics of Mexican heritage: Implications for mental health. In M. Miranda & R. Ruiz (Eds.). *Chicano aging and mental health*. (DHHS Publication No. ADM 81-952). Rockville, MD: National Institute of Mental Health.

Yeatts, D.E., Crow, T., & Folts, E. (1992). Service use among low-income minority elderly: Strategies for overcoming barriers. *The Gerontologist, 32*. (1), 24-32.

Dominican Immigrant Elders:
Social Service Needs,
Utilization Patterns, and Challenges

Ana Paulino, ACSW, EdD

SUMMARY. It is estimated by the 1991 U.S. Census Bureau that over one million Dominicans reside in this country. The growth of the Dominican ethnic group in the United States is also reflected in a steady increase of the elderly population. A review of census data and other pertinent literature identify the Hispanic population in general and the elders in particular as economically and socially at risk.

This article includes an overview of the Dominican immigrants and their patterns of immigration to the United States. A discussion about the Dominican immigrant elders follows by using information obtained from a focus group held at a senior citizen center located in an inner city of New York; recommendations and implications for practice and research are included as well. An ecological framework is used as a practice perspective and as a way of understanding and organizing the material presented.

Results from the focus group indicate the Dominican immigrant elders need services that will improve their quality of life by getting housing; getting their naturalization papers in order; and receiving medical and social services with the assistance of their social worker. An analysis of the participants' discussion in the group points to a strong sense of spirituality as a way of coping with stressful events such as an

Ana Paulino is Associate Professor, Hunter College School of Social Work, 129 East 79th Street, New York, NY 10021.

The author gratefully acknowledges the invaluable research assistance of Eva Paulino, Manny Gonzalez, and Patricia Hernandez-Kenis.

[Haworth co-indexing entry note]: "Dominican Immigrant Elders: Social Service Needs, Utilization Patterns, and Challenges." Paulino, Ana. Co-published simultaneously in *Journal of Gerontological Social Work* (The Haworth Press, Inc.) Vol. 30, No. 1/2, 1998, pp. 61-74; and: *Latino Elders and the Twenty-First Century: Issues and Challenges for Culturally Competent Research and Practice* (ed: Melvin Delgado) The Haworth Press, Inc., 1998, pp. 61-74. Single or multiple copies of this article are available for a fee from The Haworth Document Delivery Service [1-800-342-9678, 9:00 a.m. - 5:00 p.m. (EST). E-mail address: getinfo@haworthpressinc.com].

61

illness. The elders also show a strong desire to adjust to new situations, e.g., as it is evidenced by their commitment to comply with newly established welfare immigration law which regulates eligibility benefit requirements. Service providers will need to be familiar with the new immigration policies in order to be effective in providing adequate services for immigrant elders at risk. *[Article copies available for a fee from The Haworth Document Delivery Service: 1-800-342-9678. E-mail address: getinfo@haworthpressinc.com]*

Aging as a part of the developmental life cycle is experienced by Dominicans in a similar universal manner as most individuals regardless of ethnic group. However, there are certain sociocultural factors which impact the aging process among Dominicans in the United States, e.g., poverty, limited formal education, cultural values, familial commitment, nationality allegiance, and spirituality.

This article presents an overview of Dominican immigrants including their patterns of immigration to the United States. This overview will serve to understand who they are within the Latino community; a discussion about the Dominican immigrant elders will follow using information obtained from a focus group held at a senior citizen center located in an inner city of New York; recommendations and implications for practice and research will be included as well. An ecological framework will be used as a practice perspective and as a way of understanding and organizing the material presented. The ecological perspective used is grounded in general systems theory. General systems theory is the study of the relationship of interactional parts in context, emphasizing their unity and organizational hierarchy. It offers a perspective on the way in which one area of social life is related to another. It involves a system of interdependent parts in which a change in any relationship will have an effect on all other relationships (Germain & Gitterman, 1980; Hartman & Laird, 1983). An understanding and application of the ecological perspective is useful in framing the lives of the Dominican immigrant elders in the United States.

AN OVERVIEW OF DOMINICANS IN THE UNITED STATES

Dominicans comprise the second largest Hispanic/Latino group in New York City after Puerto Ricans (Georges, 1990). It is estimated by the 1991 U.S. Census Bureau that over one million Dominicans reside in this country. Dominican immigration has been mainly directed to New York City. The reason for this is unclear, but New York City is strongly advertised in the Dominican Republic as the most desirable place for immigrants to seek work. Dominicans are also found in substantial numbers in New Jersey, Florida,

Washington, D.C., Puerto Rico, Massachusetts, Rhode Island, and Connecticut. The growth of the Dominican ethnic group in the United States is also reflected in a steady increase of the elderly population. With regard to the rate of increase in the proportion of elderly persons, it has been observed that the Hispanic population will experience the fastest rate (Ozama, 1997). A review of census data and other pertinent literature identify the Hispanic population in general and the elders in particular as economically and socially at risk (U.S. Bureau of the Census, 1992; AARP, AOA, 1993; Tran & Dhooper, 1996; Hernandez & Torres-Saillant, 1996; Burnette, 1997). Given these demographics and different characteristics exhibited by three waves of Dominican immigration described below, several social service needs of the Dominican elders emerge. Social work's response to Dominican immigrants has been limited by the scarcity of personnel capable of understanding their cultures, their migration experiences, and the issues they face in the process of adjusting to life in the United States (Drachman, Kwon-Ahn & Paulino, 1996).

An analysis of the immigration flows of Dominicans to the United States identifies three distinct groups. These groups of Dominican immigrants share similar adjustment problems with other immigrants residing in the United States, but they also have unique needs and varying attitudes toward seeking help from human service professionals. For example, the Trujillo[*] era (1930-1961) group are established professionals, many of whom are too proud to seek help. The post-Trujillo era immigrants, middle-class to working-poor Dominicans, might seek help from a social service agency as a result of a referral from their child's school. The third group, who immigrated to urban areas from 1982 to 1986, is comprised of the very poor "flotilla" people and "jodedores" who might be seen in inpatient units with a dual diagnosis, e.g., substance abuse and mental illness or substance abuse and HIV positive. These three groups of Dominican immigrants have unique needs and varying attitudes toward seeking help from human service professionals (Paulino, 1994).

Within the three waves of immigration from the Dominican Republic, there is no reported data about the elderly. One view is that since the primary push and pull for immigrants to come to the United States has been driven in part by their demonstrated ability to join the work force, it is suspected that the elderly were not encouraged to travel unless they were coming on a tourist visa.

DEMOGRAPHIC PROFILE OF DOMINICANS IN THE UNITED STATES

As previously stated, a number of problems exist related to the numbers of Dominican elders in the United States. Moreover, Dominicans were not

---

[*]Rafael L. Trujillo, was the president of the Dominican Republic for thirty years. His regime ended with his assassination in 1961.

counted separately by the U.S. Census Bureau until 1990 (as a write-in category). This limits demographic information about U.S. Dominicans. Traditionally, reports about Dominicans have been included with other Hispanics, making it difficult to have a separate count of the actual number of Dominicans and their demographic characteristics. Until recently, very little information has been available on the composition of the Dominican migrant stream to the United States, but in the last few years, a body of research has begun to be accumulated. It should be added that even though the 1990 U.S. Census included a place for Dominicans to check their nationality, the figures are omitted in the 1991 published report. Dominicans are still included under the category of "other Hispanic" (U.S. Bureau of the Census, 1991). This lack of systematic recorded data on Dominicans in general and the elders in particular poses a major research barrier, as well as an opportunity, for scholars, service providers, and other professionals who wish to learn more about this population. Burnette (1997) makes a similar assertion, noting that "more data are needed on the characteristics and needs of Dominicans, whose numbers are growing rapidly in New York City" (p. 132).

The Dominican population in the United States consists of a large group of young persons ranging from 20 to 30 years of age, and women (Georges, 1990), many of whom are single parents with children younger than 18 years of age. Many families live in poverty (Hernandez & Torres-Saillant, 1996). Low or substandard wages from employment in factories, restaurants, grocery stores, money exchanges, or home care are common. In 1990, the median Dominican household income in New York City was $9,367 (personal communication, New York City Mayor's Office Staff and the Dominican Consulate, 1991). It is suspected that Dominican immigrant elders have a higher poverty rate than the younger population since their income is fixed, based on monthly SSI and/or SSA payments. The general consensus in the literature is that non-white older persons have higher rates of poverty than their Caucasian counterparts (Burnette, 1997; Ozama, 1997; Tran & Dhooper, 1996; Gallego, 1991). Dominican elders are not an exception to this socio-economic reality affecting many Hispanics.

In short, Dominican emigration, excluding the Trujillo era group, has been characterized as a politically as well as economically induced movement, e.g., unrestricted immigration policy supported by the United States and the Dominican government (Grasmuck & Pessar, 1991). Georges (1990) indicates that the majority of Dominican immigrants traveling to the U.S. were not unemployed in the Dominican Republic; instead, they have reported a desire to work and to earn higher wages as an important motive for their migration to the United States. Although systematic data are needed, it seems clear that Dominican immigrant families are a rapidly growing ethnic group with increasing needs for social services including the elderly.

CULTURAL ASSESSMENT

As noted earlier, Dominican immigrants are socially diverse, representing various social strata of Dominican society. They have experienced numerous complex socio-economic and political situations which have conditioned their overall migratory journey or experience. The idea of returning to the island, which many hold, also conditions the Dominican migratory experience. The immigration process is viewed as a temporary one. However, the reality is that Dominican immigrants live in two worlds, the Dominican Republic and the United States. It is believed that this process of circular migration is reflective of their ambivalence about their socio-political status here in the U.S. This circular migration is addressed in the literature as a transnational migrant network phenomenon in which middle-class socio-economic status on the island is maintained by the immigrants' reliance on what is described as a continuous economic dependence on the U.S. market (Georges, 1990; Grasmuck & Pessar, 1991).

In an ethnographic study conducted by Duany (1994), it was found that most respondents felt Dominican, not American and not even Dominican-American. When the immigrants described their country of origin, they often used emotional terms like *mi patria* ("my fatherland"), *mi tierra* ("my land"), *mi pais* ("my country"), and *la madre tierra* ("the motherland"). Duany also observed that respondents emphasized the possessive adjective (*mi*) when referring to the Dominican Republic, but not to the United States, which they usually called *este pais* ("this country"). This distance was attributed to the participants' desire to remain emotionally attached, almost in a nostalgic manner, to their country of origin (Duany, 1994). It has been said that Dominicans exhibit a strong attachment to their native land to the point of perhaps undermining, complicating, or delaying their adaptation to the receiving society (Hernandez & Torres-Saillant, 1996).

Dominican immigrants are active participants in political and economic affairs taking place in the Dominican Republic. In contrast, their political participation in the United States has been reported as limited. This limited participation is measured by their reluctance to become U.S. citizens. Becoming a naturalized American is a process described by the participants in the focus group with mixed emotions or a sense of ambivalence. However, they are now becoming naturalized American citizens which usually means that they need to enroll in a preparatory course which includes English as a second language and American history. For years, Dominicans as a community had a low rate of naturalization despite their steadily increased migration to the United States (Grasmuck & Pessar, 1991; Torres-Saillant & Hernandez, 1998). More recently, however, the 1980 census shows that Dominicans are indeed, becoming United States citizens. A more recent contributing factor influencing Dominicans, especially the elders and persons receiving governmental assistance to become naturalized citizens of the U.S., is associated with the new welfare immigration law which regulates eligibility benefit requirements. It is not sufficient to be a permanent resident to be entitled to state and federal programs, it is also expected that the individuals demonstrate proof of citizenship (Vialet & Eig, 1997). For instance, benefits for immigrants now receiving SSI will end after the recipient's next annual evaluation unless there is a change of citizenship. Similar requirements will affect non-citizens receiving medicaid, cash assistance, food stamps, public housing, and other social services (Parra, 1997).

When a client does not speak English, professionals need to explore the socio-political context affecting the immigration process of that individual. It may be possible that what appears to be resistance to learning English might be, instead, a symptom of a deeper conflict or fear of losing their Dominican identity, and being associated with the "dominant group." Similarly, if an immigrant shows ambivalent feelings about becoming a naturalized citizen of the U.S., human service providers must explore individual, family and immigration history which may influence the decision to give up Dominican nationality. Both issues, language and naturalization, require a thorough assessment of the effects on the immigrant's self-concept, identity, and wish to acculturate to the host society. Social workers must assess the impact of socio-political and cultural factors on immigrants' coping styles and the community resource systems which may be utilized to acculturate effectively to the new environment. Additionally, professionals must explore the nature and circumstances of the immigrant's experiences and intervene accordingly. Stressors interfering with the process of acculturation and adaptation to the host society need to be promptly assessed in order to reduce the level of conflict experienced by immigrant families and to maximize their collective advancement in the community.

A GROUP EXPERIENCE: GROUP PARTICIPANTS CONSTRUCTING THEIR NARRATIVES

For the purpose of collecting the necessary data for this study, a focus group was used, consisting of ten Dominican immigrant elders who reside in Washington Heights, New York City. Washington Heights has been identified as having the highest number of Dominican residents in New York City (Duany, 1994). Dominican immigrant elders who attend a senior citizen center were invited to participate in the focus group to discuss their social service needs, concerns, and resources known to them in the community. The senior citizen center is also affiliated with a medical clinic where most of the group participants receive medical care.

The group participants completed a questionnaire which focused on concrete demographic information. All the information obtained from the focus group was in Spanish. The researcher and an assistant served as facilitators of the focus group. One facilitator was Dominican, the other was Columbian, and both were fluent in Spanish. A focus group guide, consisting of semi-structured and open ended questions, was developed to generate relevant data identifying: who are the Dominican immigrant elders as an ethnic group; what are their issues, concerns, and challenges as they have become members of their community in the United States, especially in Washington Heights; how has their life style changed; what would make their lives more fulfilled at the present time; what has helped them to cope with life transitional events; what type of services are they receiving in their community; what services are missing which they would like to have available; what do they do when they find themselves in need of help; what are their beliefs about what helps; and where do they go when they need help?

The focus group lasted 90 minutes and it was audiotaped. The audiotape was transcribed and analyzed using a structural conceptual framework developed by Sacks (1984), Goffman (1974) and Garfinkel (1967). These authors believe that interactions and narratives can be recorded and systematically analyzed. They maintain that these recorded events provide a conceptual design reflecting a sequential ordering of 'story telling.' This type of data collection and analysis is consistent with Hartman's (1992) suggestion about the need for exploring subjugated knowledge in a manner that professionals learn from the clients' life experiences by using an ethnographic approach to data collection. Hartman (1992) encourages researchers to develop a partnership and collaborative relationship with indigenous groups in which a dialogue exists and "local knowledge" is recognized.

The audiotaped session obtained from the focus group provides a data base that is retrievable which also preserves events in the context in which they occur. Consequently, this type of research tool offers the advantage of examining interactions extensively. The group facilitators and the participants participated in the construction of their 'stories.' The interpretation of results/findings is limited by the small size of the sample of the focus group. Additionally, since the participants were members of the senior citizens center, they may not be representative of the larger Dominican community. However, a focus group was used as a method for collecting data and to provide what Hartman (1992) identifies as giving voices to "local knowledge" derived from people's life experiences. "We must enter into a collaborative search for meaning with our clients and listen to their voices, their narrative, and their construction of reality" (p. 484). This process of knowledge-building has been also addressed by Yegidis and Weinbach (1996) who suggest that when very little is known about a target issue, an exploratory inquiry seems to be the most appropriate design to begin a systematic data collection process. As indicated earlier, little systematic data are available about Dominicans in general and elders in particular.

GROUP COMPOSITION AND MAJOR THEMES

The group participants were primarily from the northern section of the Dominican Republic, an area called *"el Cibao."* The participants' length of time in the United States ranged from 6 to 31 years. There were six men and four women, ages ranging from 61 to 80 years. They all had completed an elementary level of education. Eight of the ten participants identified themselves as monolingual, Spanish speaking only. Two participants expressed having an adequate level of English fluency. Assistance in completing the questionnaire was requested by the participants although the material was in Spanish. This request suggests that some of them may have difficulty understanding and prefer this type of help in completing forms and other related documents. Their employment experiences have been primarily factory workers. Presently, they are retired, receiving either SSI and/or SSA. Two participants reported having no income. Nine of ten participants have children, ranging in ages 14 to 59 years. In this area they expressed having an adequate support system which is also reciprocal in providing some mutual aid. A significant number of the respondents are actively involved in the community by doing volunteer work through the local church or the senior citizen center. They all expressed having some health related problems such as cardiovascular problems, hypertension, and diabetes. Two participants had suffered a stroke and a heart attack. They all indicated having changed their eating habits and overall lifestyles in order to maintain a sense of "well being." For example, they have eliminated or reduced the amount of sugar and salt intake. They exercise and keep regular medical visits as a way of improving and monitoring their health.

Three primary needs emerged in response to some of the questions asked. The first two needs focused on improving the quality of life by getting housing and getting their naturalization papers in order. The third need was related to receiving medical and social services with the assistance of their social worker. They found the worker to be resourceful, compassionate and knowledgeable of their needs and culture. For example, one participant expressed that the social worker helps her to feel happy: "She is excellent; she is the best." Another participant echoed similar compliments and added that "She is a fair person who takes good care of all of us. God bless her."

Overall, the participants described their experience in the United States, and in particular in Washington Heights, in positive terms. They felt that this country has given them an opportunity to earn a living and to be able to send some money to their relatives in the Dominican Republic. The tone of their description reflected an almost stoic posture about their environment and family commitment. Fifty percent of the participants have become naturalized citizens. The others are either in the process of becoming U.S. citizens or are completing their legal papers to become permanent residents. It was also suggested that, based on the information provided by the elders who participated in the focus group, they perceived themselves as permanent members of American society, hopeful of a better future. They were very active in performing family and community activities.

When participants were asked what they would need in order for them to feel fulfilled or complete, five participants expressed needing housing as their main concern. They had been waiting for years for public housing. They added that getting public housing will help manage their financial situation better. Presently, they spend most of their money on rent; three stated that their children contribute money toward their rent. They also reported wanting to complete their naturalization process in order for them to feel more secure.

An analysis of the participants' discussion in the group points to a strong sense of spirituality as a way of coping with stressful events such as an illness. For example, one participant described an experience of being ill and asking God to heal her. She found relief in God and the good work of her helping social worker. "I am a woman of faith," the participant concluded. Two participants, who were of the Protestant faith, indicated that they gained inner strength from their belief system: "The Lord will heal me. I place myself in his hands." Another participant indicated that she finds strength by helping others through her volunteer work with the local Catholic church: "I take care of the sick ones."

Spirituality seemed to be a central theme in shaping the world view of many of the participants. It is through spiritual beliefs that immigrant families may cope when someone significant in the family is ill or disabled. "*Que sea lo que Dios quiera!*" (God's will!) This belief implies that God guides one's destiny. In this sense, these individuals might see themselves as being subjugated to nature as opposed to being the master of their own destiny. A review of the literature reveals that the spiritual dimension of the person, particularly as it interacts with the life cycle and environmental stressors, has been muted in social work practice. Cornett (1992) emphasizes the need to incorporate the spiritual component of the client's belief system into the overall assessment and treatment plan indicating that the time "has come for social work to broaden its perspective, to include the spiritual aspects of the physical, phenomenological individual in her or his environment" (Cornett, 1992, p. 101).

Lack of appropriate integration of valuable culturally specific information places the immigrant family at risk of being misdiagnosed and inappropriately served (Paulino, 1995a). Human service professionals must develop an understanding of how the individual perceives symptom formation and curative methods. Counseling services must be flexible to incorporate therapeutic interventions for those individuals who feel that God or spiritual forces guide their choices regarding decisions which they must make about their daily problems. It has been suggested by Delgado (1995) that indigenous members' participation must be sought during the planning and delivery of service phases of program development in order to increase their participation in the decision making process regarding the best treatment options available. This outreach to community participation can maximize the level of service utilization and collaboration between the community and the larger social structure. Professionals can assist the community members to see how they are active agents of the social change they seek through recognition of their cultural and belief systems. Additionally, professionals must see learning about this group's culture as an integral part of their professional development if effective services are to be developed and delivered.

The most impressive finding of the focus group was associated with their outlook about life and their present situations. The group as a whole expressed feeling satisfied with themselves and their achievements in life. This sense of self-accomplishment was measured by the circumstances of their children. The participants felt proud as parents. Their children are not factory workers, but rather professionals, employed in the nearby community hospital. Some participants made references to their children by using phrases such as "*tesoros*" (jewels). Three male participants identified having difficulty with their children in the past due to poor communication but their relationships have improved over the years. It seems that this is an area that gives them a sense of mastery and purpose as described by Erikson (1963). Around the issue of parenthood, the participants stressed the critical role and the sacrifices that they have made in raising their children in a foreign country. Their responses suggest that being a parent is a role which has given them a sense of social status in their cultural milieu. For instance, they consider themselves as important figures who can actively be involved in family matters which require decision making. It seems that from this interaction with family members, they derive a sense of respect, acceptance, and self-esteem. Some of the participants indicated that they function as caregivers in their role as grandparents. It has been noted that older persons act as resources for their families, especially in the inner cities (Burnette, 1997). Similarly, the family is the primary source of caregiving and support to older persons (Tran & Dhooper, 1996).

SUMMARY AND CHALLENGES

In general, results from the focus group indicate the Dominican immigrant elders need services that will improve their quality of life. As the older population increases in size and diversity, social workers must keep in mind: (1) older persons are generally integral members of Dominican families, often providing help and care to other family members or receiving care themselves; (2) elders also provide a sense of cultural continuity; (3) older people's ethnicity and cultural heritage may have a strong influence on how they and their families experience and cope with aging; (4) ethnicity and cultural heritage may also affect the way help is sought, interpreted, and received; and finally, (5) members of different generations within families may have different views of the nature of aging related difficulties and the best solutions to these difficulties.

In a period of adjustment, as with immigration and aging, the family as a social institution undergoes many changes, both in structure and function. Human service providers must actively reach out to the elders during such times of adjustment and crisis. Dominican elders are survivors, an affirmation that *"contra viento y marea"* (against all the odds) they have been able to cope with adverse situations. Community leaders and human service providers must advocate and assume an active role in helping Dominican elders and other immigrant families to negotiate bureaucratic organizations which are identified as stressors in the acculturation process. Social workers who are knowledgeable and sensitive to these issues can certainly function as cultural brokers for these families. The culture broker is the individual who negotiates the challenges posed by living in an ethnically diverse, sometimes hostile society. The concept of the culture broker refers to the relationships, interaction, and linkage between the individual within the family and between the family and the broader social environment. Social workers are in a position to help Dominican immigrant elders during their process of adjustment and adaptation to the host culture. Professional interventions must take place as soon as the immigrant families or the service providers recognize a need for securing therapeutic assistance.

Most Dominican immigrant elders have uprooted themselves from their familiar environment while attempting to establish new connections in the host society. Some have done well and do not need to seek human service assistance. For the most part, however, there is a significant proportion of Dominican immigrant elders, as evidenced by the high poverty rate, who, like other elders of color, have confronted multiple environmental and life transitional issues. These elders need the assistance of health and human service organizations.

To summarize, data collected for this study demonstrates that the participants engaged in a 'story telling' mechanism as a means of sharing their concerns. The facilitators became co-constructors of the participants 'stories.' Much more research is needed to inform program planning and delivery for Latinos in general and Dominicans in particular, to examine the impact of the reform immigration policies on family disruption and characteristics of service utilization. It is suspected that immigrant families will be reluctant to consider seeking social service assistance for fear of being found out about their immigrant status (or non-U.S. citizen status). Service providers will need to be familiar with the new immigration policies in order to be effective in providing adequate services for immigrant elders at risk. In order to maximize the benifts related to Dominican immigrant elders, there remains a need for practice-based research. At the present time most of the studies concerning the elder population in the Latino community have focused on three major ethnic groups, Mexicans, Cubans, and Puerto Ricans (Tran & Dhooper, 1996; Delgado, 1995; Gallego, 1991; Starrett, Mindel & Wright, Jr., 1983). Given the rapid and steady population increase of Dominicans, especially in New York City, systematic data collection will hopefully be undertaken to include this group as well.

REFERENCES

Betances, E. (1997). The Dominican Republic after the caudillos. *NACLA: A report on the Americans, 30* (5).

Browne, C. (1995). Empowerment in social work practice with older women. *Social Work, 40* (3).

Burnette, D. (1997). Grandmother caregivers in inner city Latino Families: A descriptive profile and informal social supports. *Journal of Multicultural Social Work, 5* (3/4).

Canda, E.R. (1988). Spirituality, religious diversity, and social work practice. *Social Work: The Journal of Contemporary Social Work, Family Service America, 36* (1): 238-247.

Carlton-LaNey, I. (1997). Social workers as advocates for the elders. Implications. In M. Reisch & E. Gambrill, (Eds.), *Social Work in the 21st Century.* California: Pine Forge Press.

Castex, Graciela M. (1994). Providing services to Hispanic/Latino populations: Profiles in diversity. *Social Work, 39* (3).

Cornett, C. (1992). Toward a more comprehensive personology: Integrating a spiritual perspective into social work practice. *Social Work, 37* (2): 101-102.

Congress, E. (1994). The use of culturagrams to assess and empower culturally diverse families. *Families in Society, 75* (9).

Delgado, M. (1995). Puerto Rican elders and natural support systems: Implications for human services. *Journal of Gerontological Social Work, 24* (1/2).

Drachman, D., Kwon-Ahn, Y.H. & Paulino, A. (1996). Migration and resettlement experiences of Dominican and Korean families. *Families in Society, 77* (10).

Drachman, D. (1995). Immigration statuses and their influence on service provision access and use. *Social Work, 40*: 188-197.

Duany, J. (1994). *Quisqueya on the Hudson: The transnational identity of Dominicans in Washington Heights.* Dominican research monographs, the CUNY Dominican Studies Institute.

Dudley, J.R. & Helfgott, C. (1990). Exploring a place for spirituality in the social work curriculum. *Journal of Social Work Education, 26* (3): 287-294.

Erikson, E. (1963). Eight stages of man. *Childhood and Society.* New York: Norton.

Feit, M.D. & Cuesvas-Feit, N. (1991). An overview of social work practice with the elderly. In M.J. Holosko & M.D. Feit, (Eds.), *Social Work Practice With the Elderly,* Canadian Scholars' Press.

Gallego, J.S. (1991). Culturally relevant services for Hispanic elderly. In M. Sotomayor, (Ed.), *Empowering Hispanic Families: A Critical Issue for the '90s.* Milwaukee, WI: Family Service America.

Garfinkel, H. (1967). *Studies in Ethnomethodology.* New Jersey: Prentice Hall, Inc.

Georges, E. (1990). *The Making of a Transnational Community: Migration Development and Cultural Change in the Dominican Republic.* New York: Columbia University Press.

Germain, C. B. & Gitterman, A. (1980). *The Life Model of Social Work Practice.* New York: Columbia University Press.

Goffman, E. (1974). *Frame Analysis: An Essay on the Organization of Experience.* Boston: Northeastern University Press.

Grasmuck, S. & Pessar, P. (1991). *Between Two Islands: Dominican International Migration.* Berkeley, CA: University of California Press.

Hartman, A. (1992). In search of subjugated knowledge (Editorial). *Social Work, 37*(6), 483-4.

Hartman, A. & Laird, J. (1983). *Family-Centered Practice.* New York: Free Press.

Hernandez, R. & Torres-Saillant, S. (1996). Dominicans in New York: Men, women, and prospects. In G. Haslip-Viera & S.L. Baver, (Eds.) *Latinos in New York: Communities in Transition.* Indiana: University of Notre Dame Press.

Jordan, H. (1997). Dominicans in New York: Getting a slice of the apple. *NACLA: A report on the Americans, 30* (5).

Lobo, A.P. & Salvo, J.J. (1997). Immigration to New York City in the '90s: The saga continues. *Migrationworld, 25* (3).

Margles, D. (1995). The application of family systems theory to geriatric hospital social work. *Journal of Gerontological Social Work, 24* (1/2).

McGoldrick, M. (1988). Ethnicity and the family life cycle. In B. Carter & M. McGoldrick, (Eds.), *The Changing Life Cycle: A Framework for Family Therapy.* New York: Gardner Press.

Ozawa, M. (1997). Demographic changes and their implications. In M. Reisch & E. Gambrill, (Eds.), *Social Work in the 21st Century.* CA: Pine Forge Press.

Parra, B. (1997). Immigration: New reforms make the quest for American citizenship a mission impossible. *Diverse City, 2* (1).

Paulino, A. & Burgos-Servedio, J. (1997). Working with immigrant families in transition. In E.P. Congress, (Ed.) *Multicultural Perspectives in Working With Families.* New York: Springer Publishing Company.

Paulino, A. (1995a). Death, dying and religion among Dominican immigrants. In J. Parry & A.S. Ryan, (Eds.), *A Cross-Cultural Look at Death, Dying and Religion.* Chicago: Nelson Hall Publisher.

Paulino, A. (1995b). Spiritismo, santeria, brujeria, and voodooism: A comparative view of indigenous healing systems. *Journal of Teaching in Social Work, 12* (1/2).

Paulino, A. (1994). Dominicans in the United States: Implications for practice and policies in the human services. *Journal of Multicultural Social Work, 3* (2).

Perkins, K. & Tice, C. (1995). A strengths perspective in practice: Older people and mental health challenges. *Journal of Gerontological Social Work, 23* (3/4).

Pinderhuges, E. (1989). *Understanding Race, Ethnicity, and Power: The Key to Efficacy in Clinical Practice.* New York: The Free Press.

Sacks, H. (1984). Notes on methodology. In Atkinson, M. & Heritage, J. (Eds.), *Structures of Social Action.* Cambridge: Cambridge University.

Safford, F. (1992). Working with the old, older, and oldest: Understanding the experience of aging in America. In F. Safford, & G.I. Krell, (Eds.), *Gerontology for Health Professionals: A Practice Guide.* NASW Press.

Starrett, R. A., Mindel, C.H. & Wright, R., Jr. (1983). Influence of support systems on the use of social services by Hispanic elderly. *Social Work Research and Abstracts, 19* (4).

Torres-Saillant, S. & Hernandez, R. (Forthcoming). *The Dominican Americans: Profile of an Ethnic Minority in the United States.* Westport, CT: Greenwood Press.

Tran, T. & Dhooper, S. (1996). Ethnic and gender differences in perceived needs for social services among three elderly Hispanic groups. *Journal of Gerontological Social Work, 25* (3/4).

Tutty, L. M., Rothery, M. A. & Grinnell, Jr., R. M. (1996). *Qualitative Research for Social Workers.* Boston: Allyn & Bacon.

U.S. American Association of Retired Persons and Administration on Aging. (1993). A profile of older Americans. U.S. Department of Health and Human Services. Washington, DC: Government Printing Office.

U.S. Bureau of the Census. (1991). The Hispanic population in the United States: March 1990. Washington, DC: Government Printing Office.

Vialet, J.C. & Eig, L.M. (1997). Alien eligibility for benefits under the new welfare and immigration laws. *Migrationworld, 25(3).*

Yegidis, B. L. & Weinbach, R. W. (1996). *Research Methods for Social Workers.* Boston: Allyn & Bacon.

Middle-Aged Puerto Rican Women as Primary Caregivers to the Elderly: A Qualitative Analysis of Everyday Dynamics

Melba Sánchez-Ayéndez, PhD

Research on informal support of older Puerto Ricans on the mainland and the island indicates that it is generally women who carry out the role of principal caregiver to the elderly (Sánchez-Ayéndez, 1984, 1986, 1993, unpub. data; Dávila & Sánchez-Ayéndez, 1996; Delgado, 1995). It has been indicated that when the elderly couple is still functional, the support offered by the offspring, generally daughters, is secondary in terms of assistance with daily living activities. However, when one of the spouses dies, lives alone, or his/her health deteriorates, adult children tend to assume a more active role. It is generally female offspring who become the primary caregivers. The support that these women offer and the services they render are taken for granted due to cultural definitions of female roles and family interdependence as well as to expectations of self-sufficiency (Sánchez-Ayéndez, 1984, 1986, 1993). Most studies have focused on the type of caregiving tasks, who provides the most care, and motivations for assuming the role of carer. Few have looked at equally important issues such as the dynamics involved in the supportive task, stress faced by caregiver, and the caregiver's appraisal of the situation.

Melba Sánchez-Ayéndez is Professor of Gerontology, Graduate School of Public Health, University of Puerto Rico, and Member of the "Advisory Panel of Experts on Aging" for the World Health Organization, Geneva.

[Haworth co-indexing entry note]: "Middle-Aged Puerto Rican Women as Primary Caregivers to the Elderly: A Qualitative Analysis of Everyday Dynamics." Sánchez-Ayéndez, Melba. Co-published simultaneously in *Journal of Gerontological Social Work* (The Haworth Press, Inc.) Vol. 30, No. 1/2, 1998, pp. 75-97; and: *Latino Elders and the Twenty-First Century: Issues and Challenges for Culturally Competent Research and Practice* (ed: Melvin Delgado) The Haworth Press, Inc., 1998, pp. 75-97. Single or multiple copies of this article are available for a fee from The Haworth Document Delivery Service [1-800-342-9678, 9:00 a.m. - 5:00 p.m. (EST). E-mail address: getinfo@haworthpressinc.com].

OBJECTIVES

The focus of this investigation was to have an in-depth understanding of the circumstances in which Puerto Rican middle-aged female caregivers carry out the tasks relevant to informal support. This qualitative study centered on the following research questions: (1) Why was the caregiver role assumed? (2) What are the instrumental tasks pertaining to caregiving tendered by the middle-aged women? (3) How do the female carers perceive their situation? and (4) What are the dynamics that characterize caregiving?

METHODS

Sample selection was drawn from a list of patients who participated in a study of cultural responses to chronic pain in Puerto Rico (Bates, Rankin-Hill, Sánchez-Ayéndez & Méndez-Bryan, 1994). The original sample was scrutinized and a list of Puerto Rican adults 60 and older who suffer from chronic pain due to some type of arthritis[1] and who lived in the metropolitan area of San Juan–the capital city of Puerto Rico–were selected. From these, households in lower-middle and middle-middle class neighborhoods were selected.[2] Snow-balling technique from patients and carers was followed. Participants were also asked to give the name of other frail elderly or middle-aged female carers in the neighborhood who could participate in the study. The procedure was followed until a quota of 30 was reached.

In-depth interviews with structured and open-ended questions were conducted. The Stanford Arthritis Center Health Assessment Questionnaire (HAQ) (Fries et al., 1980) was used to determine the functional ability of the arthritic patient at the moment of the first interview. The General Well-Being Schedule (GWBS) (Dupuy, 1984) was used to measure subjective well-being and distress in carers. A brief sociodemographic profile of both the carer and the older adult was obtained by structured questions. The open-ended questions to the caregivers revolved around the tasks and everyday dynamics involved in caregiving and the sources of conflict encountered in carrying out the caregiver role. Participants were also visited during weekdays and weekends to corroborate caregiving tasks. Only instrumental tasks were considered for the purposes of this study.

CHARACTERISTICS OF RESPONDENTS

Elderly Adults

Seventy-three percent of the care recipients were female and 27% were male. The median age of the elderly adult was 76; the youngest was 61 and the oldest was 87. Fifty-seven percent of the elderly had been suffering from chronic pain due to arthritis for more than 10 years; 30% for 5 to 10 years, and 13% for 3 to 5 years. Fourteen of the 22 elderly female care-recipients were widowed, four were married, two were divorced, and two never married. Two of the eight men were married, three were widowers, and three were divorced.

None of the elderly were sufficiently indigent to qualify for government-subsidized home care and neither their income nor their adult children's income allowed them to afford private home care services or live-in help. Only 30% of the elderly lived in the home of a child or sibling.

Scores on the HAQ Scale indicated that 50% of the older adults had "much difficulty" in terms of functional ability. They were followed by those with "some difficulty" (44%). Only two of the aged (6%) were completely unable to tend for themselves. Both had been suffering from rheumatoid arthritis for more than 10 years and were unable to do housework, dress themselves, stand from an armless chair, or walk.

Primary Caregivers

Thirty women participated in the study. All were identified as primary carers by the elderly adults suffering from arthritis. Ninety percent of the caregivers were daughters. The remaining 10% were sisters. The median age for all carers was 52. The median age for the daughters was 52; for the sisters, 59. Two of the sister-carers were single and looking after an older sister who, like them, had never married. The other, married, was 18 years her sister's junior and had been raised by the oldest sister, now a childless widow.

Sixty-seven percent of the 27 daughters who were carers were married; 26% were divorced and the remaining 7% were single. Fifty-seven percent of the total sample of carers worked outside the home. The majority (59%) were clerical workers in the following occupations: secretary, salesperson, receptionist, and switchboard operator. Those who were professionals (41%) were employed in the following occupations: elementary or intermediate school teacher, community college professor, librarian, social worker, and pharmacist. All of the sisters worked outside the home. All the daughters who were either married or divorced had children. The only sister to have a child was a single mother.

Results from the GWBS indicated that 57% of the carers were in moderate distress, 10% in severe distress, and 33% reported positive well-being. Only 10% of the participants expressed that they would institutionalize the elderly recipient of care if they could. All carers who had reported severe distress in the GWBS were faced with caring for an older adult with great functional disability, and had been caring for the aged adult for nine years or more. Two of these women had been diagnosed as hypertensive and one as diabetic. Two had home situations characterized by alcohol and substance abuse by a husband or son. None of the results from the sisters fell under the classification of severe stress and none of them expressed that they would institutionalize their sibling. The middle-aged women were also asked if they felt stressed in their role as carers. Almost three-fourths of the sample expressed that they felt no stress at all or not much stress. All three sisters and 70% of the daughters fell into these two categories. Self-evaluations of stress were similar to GWBS scores.

REASON AND MOTIVATION FOR BECOMING A CAREGIVER

The average number of caregiving years was eight. The carers who were sisters reported a lower number of years than the daughters (3 vs. 9). However, all the respondents expressed that caregiving responsibilities had changed throughout the years and had become more strenuous as time passed, particularly those who had been carers for seven years or more.

The primary reasons for assuming the role of caregiver were diverse. The open-ended questions differentiated between principal cause for becoming caregiver and primary motivation for providing care. Reasons cited as causing the carer to assume the responsibility for the older person were: caregiving as a female role, residential proximity, and having no one else to assume the role. Being a woman, whether being the only daughter of several siblings or the oldest or youngest daughter was closely linked as the cause to assume responsibility. The following statement is an illustration of this:

> Taking care of your elderly parents is primarily a woman's responsibility. Women are more reliable. Sons do not help as much or in the same ways.

Some of the women declared that, as women, it was their responsibility to assume the carer role. They believe that support offered by offspring or sibling is related to gender. Women are perceived as belonging to the domestic domain and held responsible for the care of family members. Some of the respondents also expressed a conviction that birth order and being female has an association to responsibility for the aged parent. Two of the women who provided these answers said:

> I am the oldest daughter and it is my obligation as the eldest. You know, men do not look after their parents in the same way, even if he [ailing father] is a man. The oldest daughter is generally the one who since youth is taught to be responsible for all and to maintain family relations.

I was the youngest of the sisters and my parents and grandparents always told me that the youngest daughter was the one who had to look after the parents when they aged.

Reasons subsumed under residential proximity alluded to migration of other siblings to different areas of Puerto Rico or the United States besides being the one closest to the residence of the sick parent. The sisters who are carers cited similar reasons in terms of their other living brothers and sisters.

The majority of the respondents stated that the primary motivation for providing care was familial obligation: filial or fraternal. Familial responsibility was closely linked to filial reciprocity and the reasons offered in terms of familial duty stemmed mainly from reciprocity. Many of the respondents were not able to disassociate emotional attachment from familial responsibility or cite one as the primary motivation over the other. The following statement from a daughter illustrates the concept of filial duty:

My father left her [mother] when we were young. My oldest brother was 13; I was 9. He [father] left for New Jersey and never sent any money. She insisted that we stay in school. She cleaned houses, ironed clothes . . . any job she could perform. How can we forget all that? We were poor but there was always food on the table. She put me through the two years of secretarial school because she wanted me, her only daughter, to have a better opportunity at life. I can not turn my back on her. It is my obligation as a daughter.

One of the carers who is a sister expressed the following in terms of sibling responsibility:

We were always close. She was the oldest of us and I was the youngest. She always looked after me and has a been a wonderful aunt to my daughter. Even now with her arthritis, she helps me look after my grandchildren. My mother raised us to look after each other. It is my duty as a sister. Besides, we always got along well.

Love was also cited as a motivation for performing the main carer's role. The concept of filial or sibling love is intertwined to the nature and previous history of the particular mother-daughter or older sister-younger sister relationship. One daughter expressed the following:

She was an excellent mother. She gave us so much love! It is not so easy to look after her now that her condition requires so much attention. It requires a lot of work. But how can I say that I love her and not take care of her? I can not be like my youngest sister who just stops by to visit.

One of the three sisters stated something similar:

> We always got along well. She was my favorite sister and I was hers despite our age differences. Since neither of us got married, we always lived together and helped each other. What am I supposed to do now that she needs me? Put her in an institution? Never as long as I am in good health! What kind of a sisterly love would that be? I couldn't do that to her. That is not how we were brought up to love one another and care for one another.

CAREGIVING TASKS

Daily Tasks

The caregiving tasks that the majority of the women expressed that they perform daily or every other day were: light household cleaning, giving the old person a bath, and meal preparation. In the instance when the dependent elderly is a father and he needs help with self-hygiene, then the mother, brother, husband, or son of the female caregiver helps perform the chore. Twenty-seven percent of the daughters were the primary caregiver to their ailing fathers. In two cases, the mother of the caregiver was alive and helped sometimes but the two elderly women also suffered from chronic diseases and were not able to help all the time in bathing their ill spouse. A male relative assisted the female caregiver when the elderly father was not able to bathe himself. Two middle-aged women expressed the following:

> My mother tries to help but she herself needs help. I could do it [bathing sick father] myself but he [father] refuses to allow my seeing him naked. . . . My youngest brother stops by every day after work and takes care of the bath. I am lucky that he lives close by and must pass their house on his way home from work. My other two brothers do not live close-by and they come to visit them every other weekend so I can't depend on them for assistance with the bath . . . or anything else for that matter.

> I could bathe him but he [father] cried the first time I had to do it. He was desperate ["desesperado"] and yelling why God had allowed him to live to have his only daughter see him naked and bathe him like a baby! . . . Now my son and husband help. . . . But it was not easy to convince him [father]. He [father] always comments that he never expected to see the day when he would be treated like a child.

The women distinguished between everyday housechores and heavy household-cleaning tasks. Light household cleaning was defined as swift sweeping and mopping of the most frequented areas in the dwelling–including the parent's bedroom–tidying the kitchen, washing the dishes, and arranging the sheets of the bed. Heavy tasks demand more strenuous work and are performed on a routine basis, but not daily (e.g.: cleaning bathroom, meticulous sweeping, mopping, and dusting of the entire house, doing windows). Those who share the same dwelling as the aged person engage in a different dynamics than those who do not live in the same household. Ana[3] lives with her oldest sister and works as a salesperson. Her sister has severe rheumatoid arthritis and cannot assume any responsibility for household chores. Ana comes home from work around 6:30 PM, performs the daily household tasks, cooks, and feeds and bathes her sister. Carmen, on the other hand, lives about five miles from her ailing mother. She is a secretary who begins work at 7:00 AM, leaves work at 3:30 PM and arrives at her mother's house around 4:30 PM. Carmen is 48, married and a mother of three children–ages 18 to 24; all living at home. She describes her daily caregiving tasks as follows:

> I leave work and try to beat the traffic jam. When I reach her house [mother's], the first thing I do is have a cup of coffee. She [mother] always has the cup ready and some cheese and soda crackers. You see, she tries to do as much as she can but her condition does not allow her to use a broom or mop or lift a heavy pan. So I sit down for just a little while and she informs me of everything that goes on in the family: who has called, who has visited, etc. Then, while we talk, I cook something . . . and make sure that she has enough for dinner that evening and lunch the next day; nothing fancy: chicken or fish with some rice or "viandas" [starchy Puerto Rican vegetables], or if not, a soup. While the meal is being cooked, I make sure that she takes a bath and help her sit on the chair inside the tub for her legs cannot always go over the edge. She cannot rub her back nor reach her feet, so I do it for her. I wash her hair twice a week most of the time. Once she is out of the tub, I put her nightgown on and straighten the bed linen. Once she is dressed, we go to the kitchen and I tidy up the kitchen and clean the mess I've made. If she feels like eating, I serve her; if not, I leave everything ready for later in the evening when she feels up to it. . . . Every other day I pass a quick broom and mop; the serious cleaning I do during the weekend. All these things take about two hours and then I go home to do the same for my husband and children!

Meal preparation takes a variety of forms when the caregiver does not live in the same dwelling as the dependent older adult. Some women cook every day while others prepare food during the weekends and put it in containers for the elderly to eat during the week. Others cook enough food for every two to three days and a few have contracted the service of home-delivered meals.

Routine Non-Daily Tasks

Other tasks are performed on a routine basis but not daily. They are rendered once a week, every other week, or once a month. Most of these activities pertain to heavy household tasks, washing and ironing clothes, shopping for groceries, medicines or any other needed item, taking the elderly for a ride or to buy clothes or other needed articles, taking the elderly to medical appointments and rehabilitation treatment, and financial management. Once again, subtle differences appear in the case of the nine elderly who reside with an offspring or sibling in comparison to those who reside in separate dwellings. For those caregivers who reside in the same household as the care recipient, the heavy household cleaning and washing and ironing of clothes becomes part of the household chores of the caregiver as the tasks are performed inside the same house. Those who do not live under the same roof as the frail parent must perform household chores in their home and in the care recipient's house which amounts to two residences. Irma provided a vivid illustration of this last instance regarding her widowed father. She is divorced, 52 years old, with two children living at home–an 18 year-old and a 24 year-old. Her daughters, 26 and 28, are married with children ranging from a newborn to a four year-old. Irma is a secretary. She stated:

> During the weekends I must clean my house and his [father's]; I work during the week. He is a man and is not very tidy. My mother was the one who always did household chores and prepared meals. At 82, I can not expect him to do what he never did when my mother was alive. My Saturday begins at 6:00 AM. I go to his home early because my daughter comes to visit with the grandchildren during Saturday afternoons and sometimes we go to the mall or grocery shopping together. Besides, he always gets up at 5:30 in the morning, no matter what. On Friday evening I put his clothes in the washer and dry them overnight. I bring everything with me [clothes, towels, bed linen] and arrive at his house at 6:30-7:00. He is already up and dressed. If I have not had breakfast at home, I have coffee and some bread. We talk and I always do the bathroom first . . . Then I put the clean clothes in the drawers, change the sheets and towels, broom and mop the floors, dust and polish the furniture. I've learned to be fast and his apartment is small! I finish around 10 in the morning and fix him lunch. I make sure that he has enough of the medicaments and any other thing he might need. Then I come home and start with the bathrooms and bed linen and towels. I wash and iron my clothes and my children's during the week. . . . I bring

him home for lunch every Sunday and he sits around the whole afternoon. He can't walk a lot . . . his condition doesn't allow it. In the
afternoon I prepare the meals for the whole week; both ours and his. I
prepare different meals for him because he is on a low sodium-low fat
diet. Sometimes he sits in the kitchen with me and we talk; during the
week we don't talk much because I'm always on the go. . . . If he needs
a haircut, I'm the one who usually drives him to the barber; if not, my
son. My brother is always busy. I'm also the one who takes him to his
medical appointments.

Routine medical appointments affect in different ways those carers who
work outside the home and those who are housekeepers. All caregivers and
the frail elders complained about the long waits at the physicians' offices and
the rehabilitation treatment centers. Yet, those who work outside the home
provided different explanations from those who do not, of how the task of
taking the elderly to medical appointments is provided. Teresa, a 37 year-old
elementary school teacher, married with two children 14 and 10, explained
how she manages to bring her 68 year-old mother to the rheumatologist for
monthly check-ups:

The physician's office opens at 7:00 in the morning; although he does
not arrive until ten or so. My husband takes the children to school and I
take her to the physician's office; it is near my school. We are there very
early, like around 6:45. I take her inside the office and seat her. Then I
go to a nearby Burger King and bring her coffee and a pastry. At home
what she has had is just a glass of milk for she likes to be relaxed when
drinking her coffee. Then I leave for school. She calls my sister-in-law
when the doctor is through with her, usually around 11:00-11:30 and
my sister-in-law picks her up and brings her home. If I can not arrange
things with my sister-in-law because she can not take off from her
office, then I must use one of my sick-leaves from school and not go to
work.

Trina, a 51 year-old community-college professor, married, mother of three
but with only one adolescent remaining at home, and a grandmother, shared
how she juggles her responsibilities as a daughter and college professor when
escorting her mother, 76, to medical appointments:

I try to fit her appointments with my class schedule. But there are times
when it is not easy and I must leave her all by herself at the physician's
office because the wait is long. This semester, I teach some days during
the afternoon and others in the morning. If the appointment is on one of
the days that I teach in the afternoon, I take her to the physician's office

around 11:00 in the morning. I make sure that she eats a snack before we leave because she will have a long wait. She also takes a fruit or something else in her bag to munch. I leave her at the doctor's office and go to work. When I finish at 4:00 or 5:00, I go to pick her up. Sometimes I still have to wait because the doctor has not seen her. . . . She and I have had to work this out because otherwise I would have to miss work. Luckily for me, my work schedule is flexible. There are other people who bring their parents to that physician and they have to miss a day from work.

Milagros, a homemaker, 56, married, grandmother of five children 10 to 2 years of age, also depicts a similar situation. Milagros helps two of her working daughters with their children: she picks the children up from school or daycare, feeds them and bathes them, studies with them, and even fixes dinner for one of her daughters to take home. Milagros' mother, 79, has severe osteoarthritis and she lives with her daughter and son-in-law. Milagros describes how she must rearrange her daily routine when bringing her mother to medical appointments:

We try to leave as early as possible in the morning. It is not easy for her [mother] because she has a lot of pain in the mornings. In the mornings she is much more stiff than in the afternoon. But I have to pick up my youngest grandchild at daycare at 1:00 and the others leave school at different times after 2:00. At times, the physician does not come in until later than usual and I have to leave her alone at the office, pick up my youngest grandchild, go with my grandchild to the office, and pick her up. I get very anxious and she gets upset and the baby gets upset. At times I find myself incriminating her. It is not her fault and then I feel awful. It is not easy when she has a medical appointment because one never knows how long the wait will be at the physician's office. Many times there is something unexpected and I get tense.

Health Emergencies

The primary caregivers also assume a primary role during health crises. When the older adult does not live with her/his daughter, the daughter takes the older parent into her home or stays at the parent's house. It is generally those who are single who stay overnight at the parent's dwelling until the crisis passes. If the elderly is hospitalized or bedridden at home, support from other family members in terms of staying during the day and overnight is frequent and a schedule is worked out, generally by the primary caregiver. However, the primary carer checks every day on things, and the other family members report to her. She is also the one who is most likely to spend the majority of the evenings with the ailing care recipient, specifically when it is a mother or sister. When the main carer works, she takes turns with other family members in terms of staying overnight with the elderly mother. In the case of fathers, a son stays overnight, or there is no one to stay with the father, as hospitals do not allow women to stay in rooms of two or more male patients. Lourdes speaks of how her oldest sister Myriam, 52 and the primary caregiver to their 77 year old divorced father, arranged the family schedule when the old man had to undergo hip replacement due to rheumatoid arthritic deterioration:

> She took care of everything; she is very good at that. She got most of us to cooperate. She even called our brother in Chicago and he came for a week. He was the one who stayed in the hospital those nights. We all helped in the best way we could. Even some of the eldest grandchildren helped during the day since it was summer and they were out from school. Not everyone helped the same but most helped in something. When he was released from the hospital, Myriam brought him home with her. She also worked out a schedule of who would stay with him when he was at her home once she had to go back to work after she used her vacation-time for the operation and the first week at home. But she was the one in charge of everything. . . . Once he was fully recuperated he moved back into his apartment.

Tasks That Demand the Most

The women overwhelmingly agreed that the three instrumental tasks that demanded the most from them were: taking the older adult to medical appointments or rehabilitation treatments, household cleaning (light and heavy), and bathing the sick (see Table 1). The responses revolved around the amount of time that the tasks require or the physical strain they involve. Those who are part of the formal labor force and reside in a different dwelling from that of the care recipient stated that the heavy housework had to be performed on Saturdays, which was the day that they use to catch up with the heavy cleaning chores at their own household. Escorting and transporting the ill elderly to a physician's appointment was perceived as taking many hours, specifically those hours spent waiting for the doctor to examine the patient.

The following are examples of the respondents' perceptions of these most demanding tasks and the strains involved. They pertain to grooming and household cleaning. Illustrations of the demands exerted by escorting and transporting the care recipient to a medical appointment were offered in a previous section. Marta, 53, divorced, mother of two married sons, a switchboard operator, and whose mother has been living with her for two years, explains the strains involved in daily bathing:

TABLE 1. Types of Care Provided (Percent)

	All (n = 30)	Daughters (n = 27)	Sisters (n = 3)
TASKS *			
Household chores	100.0	100.0	100.0
Meal preparation	100.0	100.0	100.0
Transportation/Escort to medical appointments	100.0	100.0	100.0
Financial management	100.0	100.0	100.0
Shopping (groceries and other basic articles)	93.3	81.5	100.0
Washing/Ironing clothes	83.3	81.5	100.0
Transportation other than medical appointments	80.0	77.8	100.0
Personal grooming	63.3	63.0	100.0
**MOST STRESSFUL TASKS ** **			
Transportation/Escort to medical appointments	100.0	88.9	100.0
Household chores	70.0	77.8	33.3
Personal grooming	63.3	63.0	66.7
Washing/Ironing clothes	60.0	66.6	0.0
Meal preparation	46.7	66.6	0.0

* Participants were asked to mention the tasks that they performed. No limits were imposed. Responses were then classified into the categories established by the researcher.

** Respondents were asked to name three most stressful tasks. Not rank order them. Those categories mentioned by more than 30% of the caregivers were selected.

Bathing her is difficult too. I generally do it before going to bed and am exhausted by then. I don't do it earlier because when I arrive I am tired from work and like to rest for about an hour or so; depending on what I must do. . . . I get up at 5:20 in the morning and leave for work by 6:30 at the latest. . . . I rest for a while and begin fixing dinner for the two of us. She can't lift a heavy pot. Then we both watch the soap opera and I talk on the phone to my children or one of my sisters–it depends. By that time, it is about 9:30 and I am sleepy. . . . One must be careful with her bath. I sit her on the chair very carefully. I'm gentle when bathing her because her skin is very delicate and she may bleed. Her bath takes about 20-30 minutes between bathing, drying and dressing her [mother has rheumatoid arthritis and can barely move her elbows and shoulders]. When I wash her hair it takes longer. She gets tired from all this. I can't rush her. . . . And all I want is to go to bed and collapse.

Josefina, 54, is married with two married children and a recently divorced daughter who moved in with her parents about a year ago, bringing a two-year old son with her. Josefina works as a pharmacist at a large drug store company and resides in a separate dwelling from her father. She explains the stress involved in household cleaning and shopping for food:

> I guess what stresses me the most is cleaning his apartment. The irony of it all is that I have a cleaning woman who comes in twice a week to my house to help me. But she charges a lot and we can't afford to have her another day. My daughter contributes for one of those two days now that she moved in with her son. My brother and sister who live in the United States do not help us on a regular basis and his Social Security check isn't a lot. It covers some basic things but not all. But my siblings don't seem to understand this. Luckily, his apartment is a small two-bedroom apartment. I spend one of my two days off from work cleaning his house and buying his food. We have a company deliver lunch to his house from Monday to Friday and he eats the same for lunch and dinner. But I always like to prepare him some soup in case he doesn't feel like eating the same thing twice in the same day. We bring him over on Sundays and sometimes go out for lunch. He has been very good at adapting because he refuses to move in with us. . . . But he can't clean well because of his condition and his poor eyesight. So I dust, broom, mop, clean the bathroom, and wash and dry the towels, sheets and his clothes. . . . I also change the bed. . . . I guess what I find more tiresome is that I don't like to do the heavy cleaning in my own house and that I must do his on Saturday mornings when I would love to be at ease in my house. Don't forget that I leave the house at 8:00 in the morning on Saturdays in order to be able to buy his groceries when there are few people in the supermarket. I'm always in a rush on Saturday from seven until one in the afternoon.

OTHER ASPECTS OF THE CAREGIVING SITUATION

Secondary Caregivers

The primary carers were asked to name the one person who helped them the most in their caregiving functions (see Table 2). Either a daughter or husband were mentioned as the primary sources of assistance to the middle-aged woman. Siblings were the second category most frequently mentioned. Sisters were mentioned as helping more than brothers but by a scarce margin. Others who are the primary source of help to the primary carer are: sisters-in-law, nieces, and elderly mother.

TABLE 2. Persons Who Help in Caregiving Tasks (Percent)

	All (n = 30)	Daughters (n = 27)	Sisters (n = 3)
HELPS THE MOST (one person)			
Husband	26.7	25.9	33.3
Daughter	26.7	29.6	0.0
Sister	16.7	18.5	0.0
Brother	13.3	14.8	0.0
Sister-in-law	6.7	7.4	0.0
Niece	6.7	0.0	66.6
Mother	3.3	3.7	0.0
OTHERS WHO HELP (two persons)			
Sister	23.3	25.9	66.6
Daughter	23.3	22.2	33.3
Son	16.7	22.2	0.0
Brother	13.3	11.1	66.6
Sister-in-law	13.3	11.1	33.3
Niece	13.3	11.1	33.3
Nephew	6.7	7.4	0.0
Husband	3.3	3.7	0.0
Nephew's wife	3.3	0.0	33.3

The participants were also asked about the other two persons who provided assistance when they needed it but who were not primary helpers to the carer. Not all the participants could provide the names of two persons. Only the sister-carers were able to do so. Those most frequently mentioned as providing secondary support when needed were female siblings. Offspring were the second category most frequently mentioned. Both daughters and sisters were mentioned the same amount of times in the sample of 30 women. Sons came second after daughters and sisters. Sisters-in-law and nieces arrived in third place followed by brothers and nephews. One of the sisters who is a primary caregiver mentioned a nephew's wife as a secondary source of aid.

Women are the primary components of the caregiver support networks. Sixty percent of the middle-aged carers mentioned that a female relative is the person who helps the most in the instrumental support chores pertaining to the frail elderly. Notwithstanding, 40% of the sample stated that a male relative provided the most help. Husbands and daughters were equally mentioned (27% each) as the primary sources of assistance to the female carers. Women also comprised the majority of those in the secondary networks of assistance to the female carer, being mentioned twice as often as men; sons ranked third.

Sources of Conflict/Stress

Despite the fact that all the women stated that they have a network of familial relations that assists them and that 90% of the carers had scores of moderate distress (57%) or positive well-being (33%) in the GWBS, and 73% of the sample expressed that they felt no stress at all or not much stress, the caregiving situation is not devoid of conflict or sources of tension and strain. Only two-fifths of the women stated that they are very satisfied or mostly satisfied with the help that they receive from those in their supportive networks. Fifty percent expressed that they are "somewhat satisfied" and would like more cooperation from those in the kin network. Ten percent are "not satisfied" with the assistance received.

Forty-seven percent of the women expressed that they were rarely helped by relatives except by those who they named as primary helper and that secondary helpers could not be counted on most of the time except during crises and, even then, the assistance provided was not enough. Three of the women (10%), all daughters, stated that they were mostly alone in terms of caregiving tasks because even the primary source of assistance was not very helpful. None of the three sisters in the sample alluded to being rarely helped and all expressed that they were very satisfied or mostly satisfied with the assistance that they receive from those in their supportive networks.

The primary caregivers were asked to state the three principal sources of conflict that they face when assisting the frail elder. Not all mentioned three sources but all mentioned at least two. Causes of conflict or stress were classified under: problems with family members or the care recipient, problems with employment, problems pertaining to personal or health matters of the carer, and problems related to role as main carer (see Table 3). Each category was further subdivided. Reasons regarding the role of caregiver were the ones least frequently mentioned, i.e., proper fulfillment of caregiver role and financial problems. Problems with siblings was the source of stress associated with family members most frequently mentioned. The primary carers complained that the majority of the siblings do not help with looking after the sick elderly or assume much responsibility and that there are disagreements with siblings who do not participate at all or enough in caregiving over how the primary carer is carrying out the supportive chores. María Luisa, 56, married, housewife, and daycaring for two grandchildren under 3 years of age, stated the following:

TABLE 3. Sources of Stress/Conflict (Percent)

	All*	Daughters	Sisters
A. Problems related to family			
Problems with siblings	80.0 (n = 30)	85.2 (n = 27)	33.3 (n = 3)
Problems with frail elder	63.3 (n = 30)	70.4 (n = 27)	0.0
Problems with husband	57.9 (n = 19)	40.7 (n = 11)	0.0
Problems with offspring	57.1 (n = 28)	78.9 (n = 15)	33.3 (n = 3)
B. Problems with employment	94.1 (n = 17)	100.0 (n = 14)	66.6 (n = 3)
C. Problems related to main carer role			
Doubts as to proper accomplishment of caregiving tasks	33.3 (n = 30)	37.0 (n = 27)	0.0
Finances	26.7 (n = 30)	25.9 (n = 27)	33.3 (n = 3)
D. Problems related to personal/health matters			
Personal/leisure time	76.7 (n = 30)	77.7 (n = 27)	66.6 (n = 3)
Lack of sleep/Anxiety/Fatigue	59.3 (n = 30)	55.6 (n = 27)	33.3 (n = 3)
Management of own household	100.0 (n = 21)	77.8 (n = 21)	0.0

* "All" pertains to total in sample who fall into the category, i.e.: "problems with husband" = those who have a husband, divorced women not included; "problems with employment" = only those who are employed, and not total sample of 30 carers. Total N of those to whom category applies included in parenthesis.

She [sister who lives about 10 miles from her] knows that I do the best that I can. I have a husband who is driving me crazy with his adjustment to retirement and I must look after these two babies [grandchildren]. She dares to complain that I am not cleaning his house [elderly father's] the way I should! . . . I'm not a maid! I have many things to do! Why doesn't she go over every now and then and help? She stops by just to visit. All she helps with is buying his medicines. That is not the most time-consuming chore! Neither her husband or sons come even once a week to help bathe him [father]! At least my husband and sons help! . . . My two brothers live in the United States and I can't depend on them. She is very much aware of that. . . . And even my two brothers sometimes dare to criticize from far away!

Mercedes, 51, an intermediate school teacher, single, and the primary carer to her sister, provides another illustration of this:

I have a sister and a brother who live in San Juan. They help as much as they can . . . well maybe not as much but they help. What bothers me very much is that they complain about how I do certain things. Even my sister-in-law dares to criticize! They don't understand her [frail sister] like I do. . . . Besides, they don't have to deal with the situation every day and every single hour. . . . It is very easy to criticize when you don't have to face the situation day-after-day.

Almost two-thirds of the respondents mentioned problems with the frail elder as a source of stress. Some of the female carers (those who did not share a dwelling with an elder) expressed that the elderly care recipient demanded longer everyday visits and that their schedule did not allow them to spend more hours a day in the home of the elder. Others–particularly those who work outside the home–stated that at times the frail older person expressed a desire to chat for a longer time. They also stressed that the changes in mood of the older person, specifically when she/he feels worse than usual, are a source of stress and conflict. Myriam, 52, single, a salesperson, and the primary caregiver to her 77 year old divorced father who resides in a separate household, expressed her feelings:

> There are times when he is really feeling bad because he hurts more or can't do as much–or little–as he can by himself. . . . He gets very depressed and seeing him like that depresses me. To make matters worse, he doesn't want me to leave and plays this guilt-trip on me. It works! . . . When I must leave because I have to go home to sleep, I feel really awful! I don't need that. I tell him that he should be thankful that he has his children who care for him. . . . But since I'm the one who visits daily, I am the one who is always faced with this guilt-trip and the depression.

Conflicts in the husband-wife relationship ranked third when family members are considered. Fifty-eight percent of the 19 married carers declared that the responsibilities involved in the caregiving role create friction with their spouses. Husbands complain that the wife spends too much time at the elder's house, that other siblings do not participate in the caregiving chores as much as they should, that they feel their privacy is being invaded by the older frail adult, and that the wife is frequently too tired to chat, go out or have intercourse. One of the women has a husband who is an alcoholic and this is a constant source of stress, particularly when the husband gets heavily intoxicated and he shouts that he does not want the old mother-in-law in his home. Her siblings have not offered to bring the mother to live with them and she complains that they have not welcomed her suggestion to institutionalize the older woman who is bedridden.

Of the twenty-eight women who have offspring, 57% expressed that problems with children was another source of stress or conflict. Adult children often complain that mothers are overstressed with caregiving tasks and that uncles and aunts do not share in their responsibilities as offspring. Another source of protest from adult children is that the middle-aged mother cannot always be relied on as often as needed to help in childcare tasks due to her support-giving chores to the frail adult. Adolescent children voiced that sometimes their mothers were too tired to listen to them or in a bad mood due to fatigue from caregiving tasks.

Ninety-four percent of the 17 carers who work outside the home reported conflicts between the roles of caregivers and employees. Reasons alluded centered upon stress or conflict arising from health crises or caused by bringing the sick elder to medical appointments and rush/tiredness caused by worker-carer-homemaker roles. Gladys, 51, married with two of three children aged 26-20 living at home, and a receptionist at a law firm, summarized both sources of stress:

> I get very tired. I wish that I could have her at home with us but there isn't that much space at our house. I'm always rushing from one place to another: work, her apartment [frail mother's], and then my house. . . . My workday demands a lot; it is not that easy to do what I do. Then, everyday the same: work, her place, and mine. I am very tired in the evenings. . . . I must take half-a-day or the whole day off when I take her to her medical appointments. Not all my bosses are equally understanding. . . . When she underwent surgery I used my remaining vacation-time to stay in the hospital with her and throughout the rehabilitation period. I even had to ask for three extra days that were taken off from my sick leave.

All the women who live in a separate household from the frail adult–21 of the 27 daughters–expressed that household chores of both dwellings are a source of stress. They complained about weariness due to twice the houseworkload and lack of time to rest from house chores. The middle-aged carers also declared that the built-in stress in the carer role and their other roles affected sleep patterns, made them feel tense and fatigued, and did not allow them leisure time or spare time to do their own personal things at ease. One woman poignantly stated:

> I yearn for the day when I can sleep a Saturday until barely eight in the morning or just stay at home doing household chores without having to rush from one place to the other. . . . Or just lay in bed doing absolutely nothing or reading a "Vanidades" [Latin American female-oriented journal]!

Another source of stress that emerged from the answers was doubts of the carer as to whether or not she was carrying out the tasks of support in the proper way. The ten women who expressed this concern were daughters. Some mentioned that they also suffered from guilty feelings as there are occasions when they feel resentment toward their situation as principal carers or the frail aged. The following statements provide an illustration:

> There are times when I feel angry at him. Can you believe that? My own father who was so good to me! I feel so guilty afterwards! What kind of a daughter am I to feel such an awful thing! It doesn't help at all to have such feelings.

> Everybody has an opinion of their own as to how I should divide my time. I sometimes wonder if I'm the one who is incorrect and don't know how to handle the situation. . . . There are times when I resent being the one who has to take care of everything. But immediately I feel guilty and ashamed. How can I think that I am a good daughter and have these thoughts? She was a wonderful mother, completely devoted to us. . . . What kind of a daughter am I?

The least mentioned of all sources of stress was financial burden pertaining to caregiving. Twenty-seven percent of the sample stated that being the primary carer involved additional financial responsibilities since not all siblings were willing to or could share in those responsibilities.

Wishes Regarding Caregiver Role

The women differentiated two areas which they would like to change regarding their role as primary carers. One focused around instrumental assistance in the caregiving functions to the frail elder. The other accentuated emotional needs. The participants alluded to assistance from family members and formal agencies. They stressed that they would like more help with household chores of the dependent older adult. They talked about assistance from other family members and formal home-helpers. Many stated that they would like for someone to stay with the elderly and perform household chores and grooming just two or three times a week. Others also mentioned support in transporting and escorting the elderly to medical appointments. The female carers did not express the desire to relinquish their role as main carer; they just solicited more help. Two of the three women who expressed that they would institutionalize their frail parent, mentioned that if their home situation were not as difficult as it was, they would not think of institutiona-lizing the elder.

The second area revolved around less interference and critique from other family members in terms of how caregiving is offered by the main carer. Many women stated that they would feel less stressed if they did not have to deal with the dynamics that ensue from this situation. Some also mentioned that at times they would like for the older person to understand that they have other things to do and cannot stay for long amounts of time at the elderly's dwelling or chatting to the elderly. They stressed that the aged's request for companionship when they are faced with other role demands was one of the things they would like to change as these demands made them feel that they were not carrying out their tasks properly.

DISCUSSION AND IMPLICATIONS

These findings provide an insight into the dynamics of the caretaking of frail Latino elderly, the situation of Puerto Rican middle-aged females who are the primary caregiver to an elder adult, and the role of primary carer of a frail older person. It sheds light on the sources of support to the main carer and indicates that men also participate in these networks of support (Delgado, 1995), even though the data suggest that they do not participate as much as women. The findings also illustrate the role of sisters as primary sources of support to the dependent aged. Research on Latino elderly has rarely focused on siblings as sources of support (Cantor, 1978).

Sisters reported less stress than daughters (GWBS and self-evaluation) in their roles as main carers. The possible differences in stress between daughters and sisters could be attributed to two factors. Daughters were mostly married and with more than two children–average number of children, 3. Only one of the sisters was married and only one sister was a mother–of one offspring. These elements are responsible for generating competing demands that influence levels of stress. The daily demands from a caregiver's spouse, children, and grandchildren seem to add to the "sandwich generation" situation of adult middle-aged women who serve as caregivers to elderly parents. The demands that they confront and the multiple tasks that they face in their domestic roles leave their toll on the amount of time that the caregiver has to devote to the elder person. Another factor affecting differences in stress levels might be that the daughters had been main carers for a longer time than the sisters. The length of time that the caregiver had been assuming the role was related to changes in caregiving responsibilities throughout the years. The women expressed that the support tasks had become more strenuous as time passed; particularly those who had been carers for seven years or more. None of the sisters had been performing the role of primary carer for more than four years.

The results indicate that the understanding of the role of "informal carer" is intertwined to certain issues. First of all, informal caregiving responsibilities flow from and are undertaken by the individual and can be influenced by others of kin (Twigg, 1989). Other persons related to the carer and the aged dependent affect the process of providing care (Carers National Association, 1992; Jones, 1986). Second, caregiving is an on-going process; it is not stationary. It occurs through time and its dynamics are influenced by past experiences relating to the relationship between the carer and the care recipient, the health status of the elderly and the carer, the length of time that the main carer has been assuming the role, the personality of the parties involved in the dyadic relationship, and also by structural and demographic variables. Lastly, people's lives are an integrated whole. A person does not cease being a carer to turn into something else. Roles interrelate and overlap and cause tension, stress and conflict. Main carers have to make choices due to their multiplicity of roles as social beings. These choices many times are the result of a strenuous decision and can themselves be stressful for both the carer and the recipient of care (Litvin, 1992).

The issue of caregiver stress has situational and subjective dimensions that pertain to meaning. These dimensions are rarely emphasized in quantitative research on caregiver burden. Yet, the carers' definition of their situation and its effect on their well-being and the quality of the supportive relationship are affected by their perception of variables such as: role conflict, constriction of social life, mastery of the situation, sense of competence as carer, and definitions of caregiver role as ensuing from cultural notions related to kinship as well as by personal coping strategies and the perception and existence of social support. The data also suggest that characteristics of the caregiving situation and the resources and/or support available to the caregiver bear an impact on the carer and that objective indicators of stress are not sufficient to describe the care demands and the burden related to support tasks (Zarit, 1990).

Directing attention to the process and context of caregiving adds a holistic dimension to the situation of elderly individuals who are sick or disabled. It promotes a more comprehensive assessment of the long-term care that occurs within the family. Service providers tend to focus on clients and exclude other people involved in the caregiving situation. It is generally assumed that informal carers are self-sufficient (Twigg, 1989). Their chores are taken for granted as they ensue from social relationships based on kinship and feelings. The needs and feelings of caregivers are overlooked as service providers focus on the needs of care receivers. It is necessary to expand the caregiving paradigm and continue to develop interventions to address the needs of family members caring for persons with chronic illness (Kahana et al., 1994). The issue of support for caregivers needs to be emphasized in the framework of service-delivery to older frail adults. The benefits and desirability of alternative interventions should be considered. Social policies that constrain attention to the needs of carers must be rectified. Better assessment approaches to enable families and the aged to evaluate their needs and capacity to respond must be developed. Attention should also be directed to family counseling approaches that recognize the dynamics of caregiving and not merely the type of support offered. More needs to be known about the long-term ability of primary carers to provide care and about the impact of caregiving responsibilities on the main carer and on the quality of care for the older adult.

NOTES

1. Patients diagnosed with severe or aggressive rheumatoid arthritis, osteoarthritis, and systemic lupus.

2. Home value varied from $50,000 to $90,000.

3. All names are fictitious so that the specific case provided cannot be associated with a particular caregiver.

REFERENCES

Bates, M.S., Rankin-Hill, L., Sánchez-Ayéndez, M. & Méndez-Bryan, R. (1994). A cross-cultural comparison of adaptation to chronic pain among Anglo-Americans and native Puerto Ricans. *Medical Anthropology*, 16(2), 1-33.

Cantor, M.H. (1979). The informal support system of New York's inner city elderly: Is ethnicity a factor? In D.H. Gelfand & A.J. Kutzik (eds.). *Ethnicity and Aging*. New York: Springer Publishing Co.

Carers National Association. (1992). *"Speak up, speak out," Listen to carers*. London: Issue Communications Ltd.

Dávila. A.L. & Sánchez-Ayéndez, M. (1996). El envejecimiento de la población de Puerto Rico y sus repercusiones en los sistemas informales de apoyo. In C. Welti (Ed.). *Dinámica demográfica y cambio social*. México: Ediciones de Buena Tinta.

Delgado, M. (1995). Puerto Rican elders and natural support systems: Implications for human services. *Jnal. of Gerontological Social Work*. 18, 92-100.

Dupuy, H.J. (1984). The psychological General Well-being Index. In N.K. Wenger, M.E. Mattson, C.D. Furberg, et al. (Eds.). *Assessment of Quality of Life in Clinical Trials of Cardiovascular Therapies*. New York: Le Jacq Publishing Company, Inc.

Fries, J.F., Spitz, P.W., Kraines, R.G., and Holman, H.R. (1980). Measurement of patient outcome in arthritis. *Arthritis and Rheumatism*, 23, 137-45. *Gerontologist*, 30, 580-581.

Jones, D.A. (1986). *A Survey of Carers of Elderly Dependents Living in the Community. Final Report of the Research Team for the Care of the Elderly*. Cardiff: University of Wales College of Medicine.

Kahana, E., Biegel, D.E., and Wykle M.L. (1994). Introduction. In E. Kahana, D.E. Biegel, and M.L. Wykle (Eds.). *Family Caregiving Across the Lifespan*. California: Sage Publications.

Litvin, S.J. (1992). Status transitions and future outlook as determinants of conflict: The caregiver's and care receiver's perspective. *The Gerontologist*, 32, 68-76.

Sánchez-Ayéndez, M. (1984). *Puerto Rican Elderly Women: Aging in an Ethnic Minority Group in the United States.* Unpublished doctoral dissertation, University of Massachusetts at Amherst (Anthropology).

Sánchez-Ayéndez, M. (1986). Puerto Rican elderly women: Shared meanings and informal supportive networks. In J. B. Cole (Ed.). *All American Women: Lines that Divide, Ties that Bind.* New York: The Free Press.

Sánchez-Ayéndez, M. (1993). La mujer como proveedora principal de apoyo a los ancianos: El caso de Puerto Rico. In E. Gómez-Gómez (Ed.). *Género, Mujer y Salud en Las Américas.* Washington, D.C.: Organización Panamericana de la Salud, Pub. Cient. 541.

Sánchez-Ayéndez, M. Qualitative research on the dynamics of support offered by female middle-aged women to frail elderly in Puerto Rico. Unpublished data.

Twigg, J. (1989). Models of carers: How do social care agencies conceptualise their relationship with informal carers? *Journal of Social Policy,* 18: 53-66.

Zarit, S.H. (1990). Do we need another "stress and caregiving" study? *The Gerontologist,* 29, 147-148.

Sociocultural Status, Psychosocial Factors, and Cognitive Functional Limitation in Elderly Mexican Americans: Findings from the San Antonio Longitudinal Study of Aging

Helen P. Hazuda, PhD
Robert C. Wood, MPH
Michael J. Lichtenstein, MD, MSc
David V. Espino, MD

Helen P. Hazuda is affiliated with the Division of Clinical Epidemiology, Division of Geriatrics and Gerontology, Department of Medicine; Robert C. Wood is affiliated with the Department of Computing Resources; Michael J. Lichtenstein is affiliated with the Division of Geriatrics and Gerontology, Geriatric Research, Education, and Clinical Center, Department of Medicine; and David V. Espino is affiliated with the Division of Community Geriatrics, Department of Family Practice, all at the University of Texas Health Science Center at San Antonio.

Address correspondence to Helen P. Hazuda, PhD, Department of Medicine, 7703 Floyd Curl Drive, San Antonio, TX 78284-7873.

The work was supported by NIA Grant 1-R01-AG-10444 (SALSA); NIA Grant 1-P20-AG-12044 (Hispanic Healthy Aging Center); AHCPR 1-U01-HS07397 (MER-ECE); NIA Grant 1-R01-AG10939-01 (Hispanic EPESE); The South Texas Health Research Center Subgrant #8; NIH Grant MO1-RR-01346 (F.C. Bartter Clinical Research Center); and Geriatrics Research, Education & Clinical Center, South Texas, Veterans Health Care System–Audie Murphy Division.

[Haworth co-indexing entry note]: "Sociocultural Status, Psychosocial Factors, and Cognitive Functional Limitation in Elderly Mexican Americans: Findings from the San Antonio Longitudinal Study of Aging." Hazuda, Helen P. et al. Co-published simultaneously in *Journal of Gerontological Social Work* (The Haworth Press, Inc.) Vol. 30, No. 1/2, 1998, pp. 99-121; and: *Latino Elders and the Twenty-First Century: Issues and Challenges for Culturally Competent Research and Practice* (ed: Melvin Delgado) The Haworth Press, Inc., 1998, pp. 99-121. Single or multiple copies of this article are available for a fee from The Haworth Document Delivery Service [1-800-342-9678, 9:00 a.m. - 5:00 p.m. (EST). E-mail address: getinfo@haworthpressinc.com].

INTRODUCTION

Cognitive impairment is a significant cause of morbidity in the elder Hispanic community. Kemp and colleagues demonstrated that 26% of Hispanic elders in Los Angeles county were cognitively impaired (Kemp et al., 1987). Bird et.al. reported that the prevalence of severe cognitive impairment was significantly higher in the Hispanic population of Puerto Rico than that reported in similar studies in other U.S. communities (Bird et al., 1987). Also, recent information indicates that Hispanic elders may be diagnosed at a younger age with probable Alzheimer's disease than the general population (Markides et al., 1997). In the AHEAD study, Herzog and Wallace also found that Hispanic elders had poorer cognitive functioning when compared with older European Americans (Herzog et al., 1996). They concluded that the ethnic difference in mean MMSE scores (1.29 points) may be due to socio-economic status (SES), but their study was unable to fully evaluate this issue. Thus, understanding the etiology and impact of poor cognitive function on the lives of Hispanic elderly appears to be particularly important.

A useful tool for gaining this understanding is the Disablement Process Model (Moritz et al., 1994; Nagi, 1976; Verbrugge et al., 1994) that is beginning to guide much of the research on disability in the elderly. The model specifies four stages in the main disease-disability pathway (pathology, impairment, functional limitation, and disability), along with personal and environmental factors outside that pathway (e.g., demographic characteristics, psychosocial attributes, adaptive strategies) that can prevent, slow, speed, or reverse the disablement process. Within this model, difficulty in performing basic mental actions used in daily life by one's age-sex group (e.g., short-term recall, orientation to time, subtraction) can be treated as cognitive functional limitations (Verbrugge et al., 1994). When used by other researchers, such difficulties are often taken as indicators of cognitive impairment (i.e., structural abnormalities and/or dysfunctions within the central nervous system). This approach is particularly reasonable when researchers are interested in measuring organic brain syndrome or dementia and use established cut off scores on the MMSE to make the diagnosis. However, the appropriate cut off scores in Hispanics is controversial (Escobar et al., 1986; George et al., 1991). Since the MMSE measures performance of several cognitive actions (i.e., orientation to place, registration, recall, attention and calculation) (Tombaugh et al., 1992), it is reasonable to treat the continuous MMSE score as a measure of cognitive functional limitation. In studies restricted to MAs only, this also avoids the problems associated with the relevance of MMSE cut points to this population group.

Cognitive functional limitation has been clearly associated with physical functional limitations and can lead to physical disability (Barberger-Gateau et al., 1992; Stern et al., 1992). Psychosocial factors have been known to positively influence cognitive functioning in persons with Alzheimer's Disease (Scherr et al., 1988). Higher income and educational background have been associated with higher levels of cognitive functioning (Fillenbaum et al., 1988; Scherr et al., 1988). Lifestyle factors such as occupation and health behaviors have also been associated with cognitive functioning (Dartigues et al., 1992; Scherr et al., 1988). To date, however, few studies have examined the association of cognitive functional limitations with psychosocial resources and burdens. None have examined this issue in Hispanics.

Not only are Hispanics the largest growing segment of the U.S. elderly population (U.S. Bureau of the Census, 1992), but Mexican Americans (MA) are the largest of the Hispanic subgroups. The purpose of this study was to: (1) determine which key psychosocial variables are correlated with cognitive function in MA elders, and (2) test a model (see Figure 1) of posited associations between sociocultural status, psychosocial resources and burdens, and cognitive functional limitation in Mexican American elderly. The model assumes that sociocultural status (SES and assimilation) has both direct effects on cognitive functional limitation and indirect effects mediated by psychosocial resources and burdens. In addition, psychosocial resources are assumed to have both direct effects on cognitive functional limitation and indirect effects mediated by psychosocial burdens. Plus and minus signs indicate the direction of the associations.

METHODS

Sample

Subjects were participants in the San Antonio Longitudinal Study of Aging (SALSA), a community-based study of chronic disease and functional status in Mexican American (MA) and European American (EA) elders. The SALSA sample was comprised of the subset of elderly subjects enrolled in

FIGURE 1. Posited Model: Association of Sociocultural Status, and Psychosocial Factors with Cognitive Functional Limitation in Elderly Mexican Americans

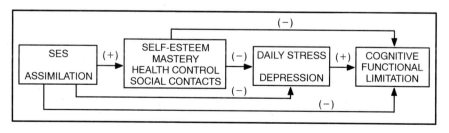

the San Antonio Heart Study (SAHS), a large prospective cohort study established in 1979 to investigate differences in the etiology and incidence of cardiovascular disease and diabetes mellitus between MAs and EAs. SAHS subjects were 25-64 years old at the time the cohort was recruited.

The SAHS sampling strategy was designed to maximize sociocultural variation among the MA study population. Subjects were selected using a multistage procedure. First, three types of neighborhoods in San Antonio, TX were purposively selected to represent distinct levels of socioeconomic status (SES) and assimilation of MAs: (1) a low-income, almost exclusively MA neighborhood ("barrio") where a traditional MA cultural orientation had been maintained; (2) a middle-income, ethnically balanced neighborhood ("transitional"); and (3) a high-income, predominantly EA neighborhood ("suburb"). Next, a random sample of households was selected in each type of neighborhood using a city directory (Polk Directory). Only MAs were sampled in the barrio since a negligible number of EAs lived in this neighborhood. In the transitional and suburban neighborhoods, stratified random sampling was used to achieve enrollment of approximately equal numbers of the two ethnic groups from these neighborhoods. All 25 to 64 year old men and non-pregnant women residing at the selected households were considered eligible for the study. Participation involved a home interview followed by a medical examination in a mobile clinic set up in the participant's neighborhood. For purposes of follow-up, only persons who completed the baseline clinic exam were considered part of the SAHS cohort.

SALSA began in 1991 as part of an NIA-funded initiative to study physical frailty in minority elderly (RFA AG-91-03, "Physical Frailty in Minority Older Populations"). Data collection was carried out from April 1992 to April 1996 and consisted of a home-based assessment (HBA) given in participants' homes plus a performance-based assessment (PBA) given at the UTHSCSA General Clinical Research Center (GCRC). All assessments were translated into Spanish using standard cross-cultural techniques and administered in either English or Spanish based on the participant's stated language preference. Data for the present study are based exclusively on the HBA and restricted to MA participants. Of the 701 MA SALSA-eligible subjects, 103 (14.7%) died before SALSA began and 3 more died after recruitment but prior to completing the HBA. Among the 595 MA survivors, 457 (76.8%) completed the HBA. There were no differences between responders and non-responders with respect to age, percent female, prevalence of major chronic conditions (i.e., diabetes, coronary heart disease, high blood pressure, stroke, and arthritis), and perceived health. But compared to non-responders, those completing the HBA had slightly more education (8.6 vs. 7.1 years, $p \leq 0.001$) and a slightly higher level of structural assimilation (stratum 2.3 vs. stratum 2.0, $p \leq 0.01$). Twenty-nine percent of the HBA interviews (131 of

457) were completed in Spanish. Six interviews were completed by proxies and are not included in the present analyses.

Measures

Demographic Variables and Sociocultural Status: Age was calculated at the SALSA HBA as date of HBA minus date of birth and recorded as the integer value for years without rounding. Gender was recorded based on participant's self-report. Classification as Mexican American or European American was carried out at the SAHS baseline survey based on a previously published algorithm developed by Hazuda (Hazuda et al., 1986) that considers the concordance (Spanish vs. non-Spanish) between father's surname and mother's maiden name, birthplace of both parents, participant's preferred ethnic identity when it indicates a distinct national origin, and stated ethnic background of all four grandparents. When evaluated against the criterion standard of predominant Mexican ancestry, defined operationally as at least three participant-reported Mexican origin grandparents, the algorithm had very high sensitivity (99.6%), specificity (89.2%), predictive value positive (90.7%) and negative (99.5%), and performed consistently better across age, gender, and neighborhood groups than did either individual surname or concordant parental surnames alone (Hazuda et al., 1986).

Sociocultural status of Mexican Americans includes both socioeconomic status (SES) and assimilation into the broader American society. Socioeconomic status (SES) was defined as an individual's location in the stratification system as determined by education and income (Haug, 1977; Liberatos et al., 1988), characteristics which allocate persons to different lifestyles and power positions (Liberatos et al., 1988). Education was measured as self-reported years of schooling within the formal, degree-granting educational system and was treated as an ordinal variable collapsed into four categories (< high school, high school diploma, some college, and bachelor's degree or more). Income was measured as household income based on earnings from all sources (including salary, Social Security, veteran's payments, welfare, stocks and bonds) of all household residents who contributed to common household expenses. Household income was also treated as an ordinal variable collapsed into four categories (< $12,000/yr., $12,000-23,999/yr., $24,000-35,999/yr., and ≥ $36,000/yr.). Education taps primarily the status (or prestige) dimension of SES, while household income taps the economic dimension of SES (Haug, 1977; Liberatos et al., 1988).

Following Gordon's model of assimilation (Gordon, 1964; Gordon, 1975), which has guided much of the empirical sociological research on ethnic and racial inequality (Hirschman, 1983; Teske et al., 1974), assimilation was defined as the multi-stage process whereby minority groups are incorporated into the common cultural life of the host society. We measured the first two of

Gordon's seven stages of assimilation: cultural assimilation (also termed "acculturation") and structural assimilation. Acculturation was defined as the multidimensional process whereby individuals whose primary learning has been in one culture (i.e., the Mexican or Mexican American culture) take over characteristic ways of living from another culture (i.e., the mainstream, European American culture). Individuals were seen as acculturating at different rates along separate cultural dimensions which may be differentially associated with discrete health outcomes. Two independent dimensions of adult acculturation were measured using the previously published Hazuda acculturation scales (Hazuda et al., 1988): Value Placed on Preserving Mexican Cultural Origin (Cultural Value Scale) and Attitude Toward Traditional Family Structure and Sex-role Organization (Family Attitude Scale). A high score on the Cultural Value Scale means that the respondent feels that it is *not* important to know something about the history of Mexico, to follow Mexican customs and ways of life, or to celebrate Mexican holidays. A high score on the Family Attitude Scale means that the respondent feels that it is *not* important for individual family members to know their family tree, to have close relationships with extended family members, to remember deceased family members on the anniversaries of their deaths, or for married children to live close to their parents. High scores on the scale also indicate a preference for equal status among brothers and sisters (Hazuda et al., 1986; Hazuda et al., 1988). Although Gordon regards all stages of assimilation as unidirectional (Pincus et al., 1989; Tinetti et al., 1988), reciprocal acculturation can occur between the minority and host cultures (Gordon, 1975). Thus, the Hazuda acculturation scales were developed and validated for use with both MA's and EA's (Hazuda et al., 1988).

Structural assimilation is defined as the process whereby minority group members gain entrance into the social structure, or societal network of groups and institutions, of the host society and is regarded by Gordon as the most critical element in the overall assimilation process (Gordon, 1964; Gordon, 1975). Structural assimilation occurs along a continuum ranging from the development of close, personal friendships with members of the host society to the establishment of primary group (i.e., intimate face-to-face) relationships within the neighborhoods, schools, and workplaces of the host society to entry on a primary group basis into the exclusive clubs and institutions of the host society, such as country clubs, elite private schools, and fraternal organizations (Gordon, 1964; Gordon, 1975). We measured the lower end of this continuum using the Hazuda structural assimilation scale (Functional Integration Scale) (Hazuda et al., 1988). A high score on Functional Integration means that the respondent has developed a fairly high proficiency in English, uses predominantly English rather than Spanish when interacting with family members and outside associates, and has a majority of close friends, neighbors, and close co-workers who are European American rather than Mexican American (Hazuda et al., 1986; Hazuda et al., 1988). Since structural assimilation is universally regarded as unidirectional, this scale was developed and validated for use only with Mexican Americans (Hazuda et al., 1988).

The criterion and construct validity of the Hazuda acculturation and structural assimilation scales have been demonstrated previously (Hazuda et al., 1988). Internal consistency of the scales among MA subgroups in the SALSA cohort (Total MA, English-speaking MA, and Spanish-speaking MA) was excellent (alpha ≥ 0.7).

Psychosocial Variables: We measured two types of psychosocial variables: psychosocial resources and burdens. The psychosocial resources measured were self-esteem, mastery, perceived health control, and social contacts. Self-esteem and mastery were measured with scales used in the MacArthur Studies of Successful Aging (Glass et al., 1995; Seeman et al., 1994; Yesavage et al., 1983). Self-esteem was measured with the 10-item Rosenberg scale (Rosenberg, 1965) which assesses the degree to which individuals perceive themselves as having positive characteristics and abilities (Rosenberg, 1965; Seeman et al., 1994). Mastery was measured using a 7-item scale developed by Pearlin and Schooler (Pearlin et al., 1978) which assesses the extent to which a person regards his life-chances as being under his/her own control in contrast to being ruled fatalistically (Beckett et al., 1996; Pearlin et al., 1978). Perceived health control was measured with a 3-item scale developed for the SAHS and SALSA which assesses the extent to which a person believes that health is a matter of fate rather than being under an individual's own control. Frequency of social contacts was assessed using a 6-item scale (Social Contacts) derived from George and Gwyther's work on social well-being among caregivers of Alzheimer's patients (George et al., 1986). The scale assesses monthly frequency of telephone and in-person contacts with family and friends as well as frequency of attendance at club and church functions.

The psychosocial burdens measured were stress and depression. Stress was assessed with the 4-item daily stress scale used in the Framingham Study (Haynes et al., 1978) and originally developed by Reeder (Schar et al., 1973) to measure self-perceived strain (i.e., the combined physiologic and psychologic reactions to personal and social situations, either real or symbolic). Depression was assessed with the Yesavage Geriatric Depression Scale (GDS), a reliable and well-validated measure of depressed mood specifically designed for the elderly (Sheikh et al., 1986; Yesavage et al., 1983). Classification as depressed was based on the standard cut-point of ≥ 11 (Sheikh et al., 1986).

Internal consistency of the psychosocial measures across MA subgroups in the SALSA study was generally in the excellent range (alpha $\geq$ 0.7). Internal consistency was lowest for the social contacts scale, with coefficient alpha ranging from 0.52 in Spanish-speaking MAs to 0.62 in English-speaking MAs.

Cognitive Functional Limitation: Cognitive functional limitation was assessed with the Folstein Mini-Mental State Exam (Folstein et al., 1985; Folstein et al., 1975), which has been widely used in community-based studies (Flegal et al., 1991; Gill et al., 1996). Following the protocol of the Epidemiological Catchment Area (ECA) studies (Crum et al., 1993), subjects were asked to complete both the serial 7's and spelling tasks. After the data were collected, two scoring methods were compared: (1) using the greatest number of correct responses from either the arithmetic or spelling items, and (2) using only the arithmetic item. The latter method was adopted because, as has been observed previously (Ganguli et al., 1990), it was less subject to a ceiling effect and increased the variance in the data, especially among European American SALSA participants. Alpha coefficients for the three SALSA MA subgroups were: Total MAs, 0.62; English-speaking MAs, 0.50, and Spanish-speaking MAs, 0.69. The magnitude of these coefficients is consistent with previous reports indicating that alpha coefficients for the MMSE in community-based samples are lower than those observed in clinical samples (Holzer et al., 1984; Tombaugh et al., 1992). One reason cited for this phenomenon is that community-dwelling subjects answer most of the questions correctly, thereby reducing the range of scores and decreasing the scale variance (Holzer et al., 1984).

Data Analysis

Sample characteristics were described using means and standard deviations for continuous variables and percentages for dichotomous variables. Daily Stress was transformed to Log10+1 in order to correct skewness and kurtosis in the distribution. Values shown for this variable in Table 1 were converted back into their original units for ease of interpretation. Relationships among the indicators of sociocultural status and among the psychosocial variables were examined using Pearson correlation coefficients. The association of sociocultural and psychosocial variables with cognitive functional limitation was analyzed using multiple regression with age and sex as standard covariates. Both single variable models, which looked at individual sociocultural and psychosocial variables, and multiple variable models, which looked at sets of variables (i.e., SES variables, assimilation variables, psychosocial resources, psychosocial burdens), were examined.

Finally, an hierarchical approach was taken to determine the proportion of variance in cognitive functional limitation explained by each set of variables and to provide some insights into the possible causal relationship between

TABLE 1. Sample Characteristics: SALSA Baseline Survey, 1992-1996.[†]

Variable (range)	Mean (SD)	%
Demographic Data		
Age (64-78)	68 (3.1)	
Female		57.6
Socioeconomic Status		
Education	8.6 (5.0)	
< 12		62.5
12		21.5
13-15		8.9
16+		7.1
Household Income	2.0 (1.1)	
<$12,000		41.5
$12,000-$23,999		30.2
$24,000-$35,999		13.7
$36,000+		14.6
Assimilation		
Functional Integration (1-4)	2.5 (1.1)	
Cultural Value (1-4)	2.2 (1.0)	
Family Attitude (1-4)	2.2 (0.8)	
Psychosocial Resources		
Self-Esteem (19-40)	30.5 (3.8)	
Mastery (15-35)	23.8 (4.0)	
Health Control (3-15)	7.9 (2.5)	
Social Contacts (0-18)	8.9 (3.9)	
Psychosocial Burdens		
Daily Stress (4-16)	7.3 (2.6)	
Depressed		22.6
MMSE Total Score (8-30)	24.7 (3.93)	
N = 451		

[†]SD = standard deviation.

sociocultural and psychosocial variables relative to cognitive functional limitation. Five models were examined: (1) demographic variables alone, (2) demographic variables and sociocultural status, (3) demographic variables and psychosocial resources, (4) demographic variables, psychosocial resources, and sociocultural status, and (5) demographic variables, psychosocial resources, psychosocial burdens, and sociocultural status. For each set of variables, only those with the greatest explanatory value based on a comparison of the previous single and multiple variable models (Table 4) were included in the analysis. Model 1 determined the proportion of variance in cognitive functional limitation explained by age and sex only. Models 2 and 3 determined the proportion of variance explained by sociocultural status and psychosocial resources, respectively, independent of age and sex. Models 4 and 5 determined the variance in MMSE net of age and sex explained by sociocultural status independent of psychosocial resources and burdens, respectively. Except for age and sex, only variables that were statistically significant in a particular model were included in subsequent models. An additional model with depression as the dependent variable and demographic variables, psychosocial resources, and sociocultural status as independent variables was examined to try to further specify the associations among the full set of variables in model 5.

Missing data on variables included in the study ranged from 1.5% (n = 7) for the MMSE to 10.7% (n = 59) for daily stress. Thus, prior to data analysis, we employed a random within classes hot-deck imputation (Lessler et al., 1992) to handle the problem of missing data. Subjects were first assigned either to a complete data subset or a missing data subset. The two subsets were then stratified by age (64-69 vs. 70+), gender, and neighborhood. This stratification produced 12 imputation cells. Complete cases within each cell were randomly paired, without replacement, with an incomplete case within the same imputation cell. Missing data on a variable within the incomplete case was replaced by a value for that variable from the complete case. A ratio of 2:1 or higher between complete and incomplete cases was required within an imputation cell before imputation was undertaken. Data were not imputed for partial assessments in which 30% or more of the data were missing. We were able to impute data for all variables in the present study for all MA subjects except the six excluded proxies.

The SAHS baseline survey (1979-1982 and 1984-1988) sampled participants at the household level and thus allowed enrollment of more than one participant per sampling unit. At the time of the SALSA study, however, 65% of participants lived in households in which they were the only SALSA-eligible resident. Therefore, no statistical adjustments were made for dependent observations within household units.

RESULTS

The sample characteristics are shown in Table 1. The average age was 68 years (standard deviation = 3.1 years), and 58% of the sample was female. Average years of education was 8.6 (standard deviation = 5.0); only 16% had attended college and an additional 20% had a high school diploma. About 40% of the sample had household incomes less than $12,000 per year; only about 15% had household incomes of $36,000 per year or greater. The average level of assimilation on all three dimensions measured was relatively low (about 2 on a scale of 1 to 4). Average scores on the four scales measuring psychosocial resources were fairly close to the middle of the scale range. About 23% of MA elders in the sample were depressed.

Table 2 shows the correlations among the five sociocultural variables as well as age and sex. The highest intercorrelations were observed among education, household income, and functional integration. The shared variance was 33% for education and household income, 29% for education and functional integration, and 29% for household income and functional integration. The correlations of cultural value and family attitude with education and household income as well as functional integration were substantially lower, reflecting shared variances ranging from 1-9%. Higher age was generally associated with lower sociocultural status, while male sex was generally associated with higher sociocultural status. However, the associations of age with functional integration and family attitude as well as the associations of sex with cultural value and family attitude were not statistically significant.

TABLE 2. Correlations Among Socioeconomic Status and Assimilation Variables in Mexican American Elderly: SALSA Baseline Survey, 1992-1996.

	EDU	INC	FI	CV	FA	AGE	SEX
EDU	--	0.575 ****	0.540 ****	0.104 *	0.275 ****	−0.096 *	0.197 ****
INC		--	0.537 ****	0.158 ***	0.238 ****	−0.116 *	0.265 ****
FI			--	0.285 ****	0.297 ****	−0.029	0.183 ****
CV				--	0.293 ****	−0.043	0.081
FA					--	−0.167 ****	−0.033
AGE						--	0.017
SEX							--

Abbreviations: EDU = education; INC = household income; FI = functional integration; CV = cultural value; FA = family attitude. P-values: * ≤ 0.05, ** ≤ 0.01, *** ≤ 0.001, **** ≤ 0.0001.

Correlations among the psychosocial resources and burdens as well as age and sex are shown in Table 3. As anticipated, psychosocial resources are positively associated with each other and negatively associated with psychosocial burdens. Likewise, psychosocial burdens are positively associated with each other. The highest correlation was observed for the association between mastery and self-esteem ($r = 0.548$, shared variance = 30%), followed by the association between daily stress and depression ($r = 0.404$, shared variance = 16%). Mastery and self-esteem were more strongly associated with daily stress and depression than were health control and social contacts. Generally, higher age was associated with lower psychosocial resources and higher daily stress, while male sex was associated with higher psychosocial resources and lower daily stress. However, the associations of age with mastery and daily stress as well as the associations of sex with self-esteem and daily stress were not statistically significant. Age and sex were not associated with depression.

Table 4 shows the association of sociocultural and psychosocial variables with the total MMSE score after adjusting for age and sex. As indicated by the regression coefficients (b) for the single variable models, each measure of sociocultural status and psychosocial resources is positively associated with the total MMSE score, whereas the two measures of psychosocial burdens are negatively associated with the total MMSE score. In terms of single variable models, functional integration explains the greatest proportion of variance in MMSE score (Adjusted R-square = 21.0%), followed by education (Adjusted

TABLE 3. Correlations Among Psychosocial Variables in Mexican American Elderly: SALSA Baseline Survey, 1992-1996.

	EST	MAS	HLC	SOC	DLS	DEP	AGE	SEX
EST	--	0.548 ****	0.296 ****	0.185 ****	−0.267 ****	−0.300 ****	−0.131 **	0.052
MAS		--	0.224 ****	0.076	−0.344 ****	−0.325 ****	−0.012	0.152 **
HLC			--	0.119 *	−0.184 ****	−0.177 ***	−0.103 *	0.183 ****
SOC				--	−0.131 **	−0.119 *	−0.098 *	−0.187 ****
DLS					--	0.404 ****	−0.037	−0.120 *
DEP						--	0.046	−0.077
AGE							--	0.017
SEX								--

Abbreviations: EST = self-esteem, MAS = mastery, HLC = health control, SOC = social contacts, DLS = daily stress, DEP = depressed mood. P-values: * $\leq$ 0.05, ** $\leq$ 0.01, *** $\leq$ 0.001, **** $\leq$ 0.0001.

TABLE 4. Association of Sociocultural and Psychosocial Variables with the MMSE Total Score After Adjustments for Age and Sex: SALSA Baseline Survey, 1982-1996.[†]

Variable and model	b	SEb	T-statistic	Adjusted R-square (%)
Socioeconomic status				
Single variable models				
Education	1.87	0.18	10.46	18.1
Household Income	1.32	0.16	8.10	11.7
Multiple variable model				
Education	1.49	0.21	7.06	
Household Income	0.81	0.18	3.28	19.7
Assimilation				
Single variable models				
Functional Integration	1.64	0.14	11.48	21.0
Cultural Value	0.65	0.17	3.79	2.7
Family Attitude	1.30	0.23	5.63	6.0
Multiple variable model				
Functional Integration	1.50	0.15	9.82	
Cultural Value	0.08	0.16	0.51	
Family Attitude	0.59	0.22	2.62	22.0
Psychosocial Resources				
Single variable models				
Self-Esteem	0.31	0.04	7.03	9.1
Mastery	0.26	0.04	5.90	6.6
Health Control	0.55	0.07	8.16	11.9
Social Contacts	0.19	0.46	4.12	3.2
Multiple variable model				
Self-Esteem	0.15	0.05	2.90	
Mastery	0.11	0.48	2.33	
Health Control	0.42	0.07	6.23	
Social Contacts	0.11	0.04	2.50	16.2
Psychosocial Burdens				
Single variable models				
Daily Stress (log)	−5.02	1.19	−4.23	3.5
Depression	−2.32	0.41	−5.61	5.9
Multiple variable model				
Daily Stress (log)	−2.84	1.27	−2.23	
Depression	−1.92	0.45	−4.27	6.7

[†]Adjusted R-square is the value obtained after partialing out the variance explained by age and sex (7.3%). T-statistics ≥ 1.96 are significant at p ≤ 0.05.

R-square = 18.1%). Among the psychosocial variables, health control explains the greatest proportion of variance in MMSE score (Adjusted R-square = 11.9%), followed by self-esteem (Adjusted R-square = 9.1%). In terms of the four multiple variable models (socioeconomic status, assimilation, psychosocial resources, and psychosocial burdens), assimilation explains 22.0% of the variance in total MMSE score, socioeconomic status explains 19.7%, psychosocial resources 16.2%, and psychosocial burdens 6.7%. A comparison of the single and multiple variable models within sets suggests that (1) most of the shared variance between SES and MMSE can be accounted for by education, (2) most of the shared variance between assimilation and MMSE can be accounted for by functional integration, and (3) most of the shared variance between psychosocial burdens and MMSE can be accounted for by depression. Therefore, in later hierarchical models examining mediators of the association between sociocultural status and cognitive functional limitation, only education and functional integration are included as indicators of sociocultural status, and only depression is included as an indicator of psychosocial burdens.

Age- and sex-adjusted associations between the sociocultural and psychosocial variables are shown in Table 5. Higher sociocultural status is consistently associated with higher psychosocial resources and lower psychosocial burdens. The strongest associations are observed for health control (Adjusted R-square: EDU = 18.4%; INC = 14.0%, FI = 17.2%, CV= 1.5%, FA = 9.0%) and self-esteem (Adjusted R-square: EDU = 11.2%, INC = 13.5%, FI = 12.4%, CV = 1.5%, and FA = 2.8%). The associations of sociocultural status with social contacts and psychosocial burdens are much weaker, with shared variances ranging from 0.0-3.5%. In addition, cultural values and family attitude appear to be very weakly associated with psychosocial resources and burdens, with the single exception of the fairly strong association between family attitude and health control.

Table 6 presents five hierarchical models examining the associations between demographic variables, psychosocial resources and burdens, sociocultural status, and cognitive functional limitation. As shown in Model 1, age and sex explain 7.8% of the variance in the total MMSE score. In Model 2, sociocultural status (education and Functional Integration) explains an additional 22.3% of the variance in total MMSE score independently of age and sex. When psychosocial resources are added to age and sex in Model 3, the total explained variance is 25.3%, with psychosocial resources explaining 17.5% of the variance in MMSE score independently of age and sex. All four of the psychosocial resources make independent contributions to the model, but health control is most strongly associated with MMSE score. In Model 4, education and functional integration are added to Model 3 to determine the extent to which psychosocial resources mediate the association of sociocul-

TABLE 5. Association of Sociocultural Status with Psychosocial Variables in Mexican American Elderly Adjusted for Age and Sex: SALSA Baseline Survey, 1992-1996.[†]

Sociocultural and Psychosocial Variables	b	SE_b	T-statistic	Adjusted R-square (%)
Education (EDU)				
Self-Esteem	1.45	0.19	7.64	11.2
Mastery	1.04	0.20	5.09	5.2
Health Control	1.22	0.12	10.33	18.4
Social Contacts	0.56	0.20	2.81	1.4
Daily Stress (log)	−0.07	0.01	−2.20	0.9
Depression	−0.09	0.02	−4.00	3.2
Household Income (INC)				
Self-Esteem	1.39	0.16	8.50	13.5
Mastery	1.03	0.18	5.80	6.7
Health Control	0.93	0.11	8.78	14.0
Social Contacts	0.43	0.18	2.44	1.0
Daily Stress (log)	−0.02	0.01	−2.54	1.5
Depression	−0.08	0.02	−4.08	3.3
Functional Integration (FI)				
Self-Esteem	1.24	0.15	8.12	12.4
Mastery	0.74	0.17	4.42	3.9
Health Control	0.96	0.10	9.94	17.2
Social Contacts	0.69	0.16	4.26	3.5
Daily Stress (log)	−0.02	0.01	−3.28	2.1
Depression	−0.09	0.02	−5.14	5.3
Cultural Values (CV)				
Self-Esteem	0.50	0.18	2.86	1.5
Mastery	0.41	0.18	2.26	0.9
Health Control	0.32	0.11	2.84	1.5
Social Contacts	0.02	0.18	0.12	0.0
Daily Stress (log)	0.00	0.01	0.06	0.0
Depression	−0.01	0.02	−0.70	0.0
Family Attitude (FA)				
Self-Esteem	0.89	0.24	3.75	2.8
Mastery	0.72	0.25	2.88	1.6
Health Control	1.03	0.15	6.89	9.0
Social Contacts	0.05	0.24	0.20	0.0
Daily Stress (log)	−0.01	0.01	−1.42	0.3
Depression	−0.03	0.03	−1.24	0.1

[†]Adjusted R-square is the value obtained after partialing out the variance explained by age and sex. T-statistics ≥ 1.96 are statistically significant at $p \leq 0.05$.

TABLE 6. Association of Demographic Variables, Psychosocial Resources, Psychosocial Burdens and Sociocultural Status with MMSE Total Score: SALSA Baseline Survey, 1992-1996.[†]

Model and variables	b	SEb	T	Incr R^2 (%)	Adjusted R-square (%)
Model 1: Demographics					
Age	−0.29	0.06	−5.02		
Sex	1.31	0.36	3.62		7.8
Model 2: Demographics and Sociocultural Status					
Age	−0.20	0.05	−4.03		
Sex	0.26	0.31	0.82	7.8	
Education	1.29	0.19	6.81		
Functional Integration	0.79	0.16	4.83	22.3	30.1
Model 3: Demographics and Psychosocial Resources					
Age	−0.21	0.05	−4.03		
Sex	0.86	0.34	2.53	7.8	
Self-Esteem	0.15	0.05	2.90		
Mastery	0.11	0.48	2.33		
Health Control	0.42	0.07	6.23		
Social Contacts	0.11	0.04	2.50	17.5	25.3
Model 4: Demographics, Psychosocial Resources + Sociocultural Status					
Age	−0.22	0.05	−4.50		
Sex	0.40	0.32	1.26	7.8	
Self-Esteem	0.04	0.05	0.84		
Mastery	0.11	0.04	2.39		
Health Control	0.17	0.07	2.41		
Social Contacts	0.07	0.04	1.84	17.5	
Education	0.85	0.20	4.16		
Functional Integration	0.93	0.17	5.55	10.6	35.9
Model 5: Demographics, Psychosocial Resources, Psychosocial Burdens, Sociocultural Status					
Age	−0.23	0.05	−4.74		
Sex	0.24	0.31	0.77	7.8	
Mastery	0.11	0.04	2.60		
Health Control	0.17	0.07	2.53	15.6	
Depression	−0.90	0.38	2.37	2.0	25.4
Education	0.86	0.20	4.25		
Functional Integration	0.95	0.17	5.71	0.117	0.371

[†]T-statistics ≥ 1.96 are statistically significant at p ≤ 0.05.

tural status with total MMSE score. The variance in total MMSE score explained by Model 3 increases to 35.9%, with education and functional integration explaining an additional 10.6% of the variance independently of the demographic variables and psychosocial resources. After introducing sociocultural factors in Model 3, the contribution to the model made by psychosocial resources remains statistically significant only for mastery (T-statistic = 2.39) and Health Control (T-statistic = 2.41). Further, the magnitude of the association between the latter variables and the MMSE score is reduced, particularly for health control. Comparing the variance attributed to sociocultural status in models 2 and 4 indicates that psychosocial resources (primarily mastery and health control) account for approximately 50% of the shared variance between sociocultural status and MMSE score (variance in Model 3–variance in Model 4 = 22.3%-10.6% = 11.7% reduction in explained variance attributable to education and functional integration). These results suggest that sociocultural status has a direct effect on MMSE score as well as an indirect effect through the pathway of the psychosocial resources of mastery and health control.

In Model 5, psychosocial burden (i.e., depression) is stepped into the model after psychosocial resources and before the two sociocultural status variables. This new model explains 37.1% of the variance in MMSE score. The two psychosocial resource variables explain 15.6% of the variance independently of age and sex, only 2% less than the variance explained by all four psychosocial variables included in Model 4. Depression is significantly associated with MMSE score. Although it only explains 2% of the variance, presence of depression is related to almost a 1 point decrease in total MMSE score. Sociocultural status variables continue to have a strong effect on MMSE score independently of the other variables in Model 5. A one stratum increase in educational level is associated with an increase of 0.86 points in MMSE score, and a corresponding increase in level of functional integration is associated with a 0.89 point increase in MMSE score. Thus, an MA elder in the highest stratum of both education and functional integration compared to an MA elder in the lowest stratum of both education and functional integration would be predicted to score 5.25 points higher on the MMSE (3*0.86 + 3*0.89 = 5.25). As with Model 4, Model 5 suggests that sociocultural status has additional indirect effects on MMSE via the pathway of psychosocial resources and, to a lesser extent, psychosocial burdens.

In order to further elucidate the associations among the full set of variables in Model 5, we regressed depression on psychosocial resources and sociocultural status adjusting for age and sex. The final model of the association of sociocultural status with MMSE consistent with the full set of analyses is shown in Figure 2. Education has direct effects on mastery, health control, and the MMSE score, with indirect effects on MMSE mediated by mastery, health control, and depression. Functional integration has direct effects on both psychosocial resources and depression as well as MMSE score and indirect effects on MMSE mediated by the psychosocial resources and burden. Health control has a direct effect on MMSE score but not on depression. Mastery has a direct effect on MMSE score as well as an indirect effect mediated by depression. Plus and minus signs indicate the direction of the associations.

DISCUSSION

Little research attention has been directed toward examining the role of psychosocial factors in the development of cognitive functional limitation among the elderly. Using the Disablement Process model as a framework, we examined the association of psychosocial factors outside the main disease-disability pathway with cognitive function in a community-dwelling cohort of MA elders. In view of the increased sociocultural heterogeneity among the MA population, we also examined the association between sociocultural status of MA elderly (SES and assimilation) relative to both cognitive function and potentially related psychosocial factors.

The results indicate that MA elders with low educational levels and/or low levels of assimilation are not only at increased risk of cognitive functional limitation, but have lower levels of psychosocial resources that may help prevent or slow down cognitive functional limitation. They also appear to have higher levels of psychosocial burdens that may trigger or accelerate cognitive functional limitations. Moreover, the results obtained with our hierarchical models indicate that both higher education and greater functional

FIGURE 2. Final Model: Association of Sociocultural Status and Psychosocial Factors with Cognitive Functional Limitation in Elderly Mexican Americans–SALSA Baseline Survey, 1992-1996

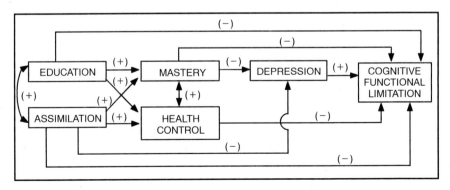

integration into the broader society have not only large direct effects on cognitive functional limitation, but also indirect effects that operate through the pathways of psychosocial resources (i.e., mastery and health control) and, secondarily, psychosocial burden (depression).

Our results concerning the association of psychosocial resources with cognitive function are consistent with those of Silberman and colleagues who found that elders who could not count on the presence of a confidant had impaired cognition (Silberman et al., 1995). Other studies, however, have found no relationship between psychosocial support and cognitive impairment (Incalzi et al., 1992; Steen et al., 1987), and one study indicated that higher education is associated with higher stress which, in turn, led to lower cognitive function (Freidl et al., 1996). It has been hypothesized that education could be a marker for lower social support in elders with cognitive functional limitation due to vascular dementia (Gorelick et al., 1993). Given our results, however, it appears more likely that higher levels of daily stress and greater fatalism about personal control over health are related to the isolation experienced by MA elders who are more likely to be monolingual Spanish-speakers and live in monolingual Spanish-speaking households (i.e., less functionally integrated into the broader American society). Depression, which was associated with daily stress and health fatalism in our study, may also be directly related to greater cognitive functional limitations.

Social workers and other community providers should be aware of the constellation of psychosocial resources and burdens that may be related to the cognitive function of MA elders whose context of daily living differs according to their educational background and level of functional integration into the broader American society. Interventions designed to increase psychosocial resources, such as mastery and health control, as well as those directed toward limiting or preventing the psychosocial burdens of depression, may also provide major benefits in terms of improved cognitive function.

It must be cautioned, however, that the present study is greatly limited by its cross-sectional nature. The "causal" inferences that we have made about the direction of the associations between cognitive functional limitation and psychosocial resources and burdens (see Figures 1 and 2) cannot be clearly established with cross-sectional data. Prospective studies are needed to determine whether the psychosocial variables we've examined: (1) lead to or prevent cognitive functional limitation, (2) result from cognitive functional limitation, or (3) simply co-exist with cognitive functional limitations. Future research should focus also on developing structural equation models which more carefully test and define the specific pathways linking discrete sociocultural variables, psychosocial resources, psychosocial burdens, and cognitive functional limitation in MA and other elders.

REFERENCES

Barberger-Gateau, P., Commenges, D., Gagnon, M., Letennuer, L., Sauvel, C., & Dartigues, J. (1992). Instrumental activities of daily living as a screening tool for cognitive impairment and dementia in elderly community dwellers. *J Am Geriatr Soc, 40*, 1129-1134.

Beckett, L.A., Brock, D.B., Lemke, J.H., Mendes de Leon, C.F., Guralnik, J.M., Fillenbaum, G.G., Branch, L.G., Wetle, T.T., & Evans, D.A. (1996). Analysis of change in self-reported physical functions among older persons in four population studies. *Am J Epidemiol, 143*, 766-778.

Bird, H.R., Canino, G., Rubio-Stipec, M., & Shrout, P. (1987). Use of the Mini-mental State Examination in a probability sample of a Hispanic population. *J Nerv Ment Dis, 175*, 731-737.

Crum, R.M., Anthony, J.C., Bassett, S.S., & Folstein, M.F. (1993). Population-based norms for the Mini-Mental State Examination by age and education level. *JAMA, 269*(18), 2386-2391.

Dartigues, J.F., Gagnon, M., & Letenneur, L. (1992). Principal lifetime occupation and cognitive impairment in a French elderly cohort (PLAQUID). *Am J Epidemol, 1135*, 981-988.

Escobar, J.I., Burnam, A., Karno, M., Forsythe, A., Landsverk, J., & Golding, J.M. (1986). Use of the Mini-Mental State Examination (MMSE) in a community population of mixed ethnicity: Cultural and linguistic artifacts. *J Nerv Ment Dis, 174*(10), 607-614.

Fillenbaum, G.G., Hughes, D.C., Heyman, A., et al. (1988). Relationship of health and demographic characteristics to Mini-Mental State examination score among community residents. *Psychol Med, 18*, 719-726.

Flegal, K.M., Ezzati, T.M., Harris, M.I., Haynes, S.G., Juarez, R.Z., Knowler, W.C., Perez-Steble, E.J., & Stern, M.P. (1991). Prevalence of diabetes in Mexican Americans, Cubans, and Puerto Ricans for the Hispanic Health and Nutrition Examination Survey, 1982-1984. *Diabetes Care, 14*(Suppl. 3), 628-638.

Folstein, M.F., Anthony, J.C., Parhad, I., Duffy, B., & Gruenberg, E.M. (1985). The meaning of cognitive impairment in the elderly. *J Am Geriatr Soc, 33*, 228-235.

Folstein, M.F., Folstein, S.E., & McHugh, P.R. (1975). "Mini-Mental State," a practical method for grading the cognitive state of patients for the clinician. *J Psychiatr Res, 12*, 189-198.

Freidl, W., Schmidt, R., Stronneger, W.J., Irmler, A., Reinhart, B., & Koch, M. (1996). Mini-Mental State Examination: influence of sociodemographic, environmental and behavioral factors, and vascular risk factors. *J Clin Epidemiol, 49*, 73-78.

Ganguli, M., Ratcliff, G., Huff, J., Belle, S., Kancel, M.J., Fischer, L., & Kuller, L.H. (1990). Serial sevens versus world backwards: a comparison of the two measures of attention from the MMSE. *J Geriatr Psychiatry Neurol, 3*(4), 203-207.

George, L.K., & Gwyther, L.P. (1986). Caregiver well-being: a multidimensional examination of family caregivers of demented adults. *Gerontologist, 26*, 253-259.

George, L.K., Landerman, R., Blazer, D.G., & Anthony, J.C. (1991). Cognitive Impairment. In L. N. Robins & D. A. Regier (Eds.), *Psychiatric Disorders in*

America: The Epidemiologic Catchment Area Study. (pp. 291-327). New York, NY: The Free Press, Inc.

Gill, T.M., Williams, C.S., Richardson, E.D., & Tinetti, M.E. (1996). Impairments in physical performance and cognitive status as predisposing factors for functional dependence among nondisabled older persons. *J Gerontol A Biol Sci Med Sci, 51A*(6), M283-M288

Glass, T.A., Seeman, T.E., Herzog, A.R., Kahn, R., & Berkman, L.F. (1995). Change in productive activity in late adulthood: MacArthur Studies of Successful Aging. *J Gerontol B Psychol Sci Soc Sci, 50B*(2), S65-S76

Gordon, M.M. (1964). *Assimilation in American Life.* New York: Oxford University Press.

Gordon, M.M. (1975). Toward a general theory of racial and ethnic group relations. In N. Glazer & D. P. Moynihan (Eds.), *Ethnicity: Theory and experience.* (pp. 84-110). Cambridge, MA: Harvard University Press.

Gorelick, P.B., Brody, J., Cohen, D., Freels, S., Levy, P., Dollear, W., Forman, H., & Harris, Y. (1993). Risk factors for dementia associated with multiple cerebral infarcts: a case-control analysis in predominantly African American hospital based patients. *Arch Neurol, 50*, 714-720.

Haug, M.R. (1977). Measurement in social stratification. In A. Inkeles, J. Coleman, & N. Smelser (Eds.), *Annual Review of Sociology.* (pp. 51-77). Palo Alto, CA: Annual Reviews, Inc.

Haynes, S.G., Levine, S., Scotch, N., Feinleib, M., & Kannel, W.B. (1978). The relationship of psychosocial factors to coronary heart disease in the Framingham Study. I. Methods and risk factors. *Am J Epidemiol, 107*(5), 362-383.

Hazuda, H.P., Comeaux, P.J., Stern, M.P., Haffner, S.M., Eifler, C.W., & Rosenthal, M. (1986). A comparison of three indicators for identifying Mexican Americans in epidemiologic research: Methodological findings from the San Antonio Heart Study. *Am J Epidemiol, 123*, 96-112.

Hazuda, H.P., Haffner, S.M., & Stern, M.P. (1988). Acculturation and assimilation among Mexican Americans: Scales and population-based data. *Soc Sci Quarterly, 69*(3), 687-705.

Herzog, A.R., & Wallace, R.B. (1996). Measures of cognitive functioning in the AHEAD study. *J Gerontol B Psychol Sci Soc Sci, 52B*(special issue), 37-48.

Hirschman, C. (1983). America's melting pot reconsidered. *Ann Soc Rev, 9*, 397-423.

Holzer, C.E.I., Tischler, G.L., Leaf, P.J., et al. (1984). An epidemiologic assessment of cognitive impairment in a community population. In J. R. Greenly (Ed.), *Research in Community Mental Health, Volume 4*, (pp. 3-32). London: JAI Press.

Incalzi, R.A., Marra, C., Gemma, A., Capparella, O., & Carbonin, P.U. (1992). Unrecognized dementia: sociodemographic correlates. *Aging Clin Exp Res, 4*, 327-332.

Kemp, B.J., Staples, F., & Lopez-Aqueres, W. (1987). Epidemiology of depression and dysphoria in our elderly Hispanic population: prevalence and correlates. *J Am Geriatr Soc, 35*, 920-926.

Lessler, J.T., & Kalsbeek, W.D. (1992). *Nonsampling error in surveys.* NY: John Wiley & Sons.

Liberatos, P., Link, B.G., & Kelsey, J.L. (1988). The measurement of social class in epidemiology. *Epidemiolgic Reviews, 10*, 87-121.

Markides, K.S., Rudkin L, Angel R.J., & Espino. (1997). Health Status of Hispanic elderly in the United States. In Martin L.G., Soldo B.J., & Foote K.A. (Eds.), *Racial and ethnic differences in late life in the health of older Americans.* (pp. 285-300). Washington, D.C., National Academy of Sciences.

Moritz, D.J., Ostfeld, A.M., Blazer, D.G., Curb, J.D., Taylor, J.O., & Wallace, R.B. (1994). The health burden of diabetes for the elderly in four communities. *Public Health Reports, 109*(6), 782-790.

Nagi, S.Z. (1976). An epidemiology of disability among adults in the United States. *The Milbank Quarterly, 54*, 439-467.

Pearlin, L.I., & Schooler, C. (1978). The structure of coping. *Journal of Health and Social Behavior, 10*, 2-21.

Pincus, T., Callahan, L.F., Brooks, R.H., Fuchs, H.A., Olsen, N.J., & Kaye, J.J. (1989). Self-report questionnaire scores in rheumatoid arthritis compared with traditional physical, radiographic, and laboratory measures. *Ann Intern Med, 110*, 259-266.

Rosenberg, M. (1965). *Society and the Adolescent Self-Image.* Princeton: Princeton University Press.

Schar, M., Reeder, L.G., & Dirken, J.M. (1973). Stress and cardiovascular health: an international study–II. The male population. *Soc Sci Med, 7*, 585-603.

Scherr, P.A., Albert, M.S., Funkenstein, H., & et al. (1988). Correlates of cognitive function in an elderly community population. *Am J Epidemiol, 128*, 1084-1101.

Seeman, T.E., Charpentier, P.A., Berkman, L.F., Tinetti, M.E., Guralnik, J.M., Albert, M., Blazer, D., & Rowe, J.W. (1994). Predicting changes in physical performance in a high-functioning elderly cohort: MacArthur Studies of Successful Aging. *J Gerontol A Biol Sci Med Sci, 49*, M97-M108.

Sheikh, J.I., & Yeseavage, J.A. (1986). Geriatric Depression Scale (GDS): Recent evidence and development of a shorter version. *Clin Gerontologist, 5*(1/2), 165-173.

Silberman, C., Souza, C., Wilhems, F., Kipper, L., Wu, V., Diogo, C., Schmitz, M., Stein, A., & Chaves, M. (1995). Cognitive deficit and depressive symptoms in a community group of elderly people: a preliminary study. *Rev Saude Publica, 29*, 444-450.

Steen, G., Hagberg, B., Johnson, G., & Steen, B. (1987). Cognitive function, cognitive style and life satisfaction in a 68-year old male population. *Compr Gerontol B, 1*, 54-61.

Stern, Y., Andrews, H., Pittman, J., Sano, M., Tatemichi, T., Lantigua, R., & Mayeux, R. (1992). Diagnosis of dementia in a heterogenous population: development of a neuropsychologicial paradigm-based diagnosis of dementia and quantified correction for the effects of education. *Arch Neurol, 49*, 453-460.

Teske, R.H.C., & Nelson, B.H. (1974). Acculturation and assimilation: a clarification. *Am Ethnologist, 1*, 351-367.

Tinetti, M.E., & Ginter, S.F. (1988). Identifying mobility dysfunctions in elderly patients: standard neuromuscular examination or direct assessment. *JAMA, 259*, 1190-1193.

Tombaugh, T.N., & McIntyre, N.J. (1992). The Mini-Mental State Examination: A comprehensive review. *J Am Geriatr Soc, 40*(9), 922-935.

U.S. Bureau of the Census. (1992). *Sixty-Five Plus in America.* (P23-178 ed.). Washington, DC: U.S. Government Printing Office.

Verbrugge, L.M., Reoma, J.M., & Gruber-Baldini, A.L. (1994). Short-term dynamics of disability and well-being. *Journal of Health and Social Behavior, 35,* 97-117.

Yesavage, J.A., & Brink, T.L. (1983). Development and validation of a geriatric depression screening scale: a preliminary report. *J Psychiatr Res, 17,* 37-49.

Challenges to Treating
the Elderly Latino Substance Abuser:
A Not So Hidden Research Agenda

Barbara Lynn Kail, PhD
Mario DeLaRosa, PhD

INTRODUCTION

The twenty-first century brings many challenges to the practitioner who wishes to address substance abuse among Latinos over the age of sixty in a culturally competent manner. This paper seeks to address these issues by: (1) Synthesizing the limited data available on the use and misuse of alcohol and other psychoactive drugs among Latino elderly living in the United States, including incidence, prevalence, patterns of use, etiology and consequences; (2) Addressing the difficulties in identifying and assessing substance abuse among this population; (3) Suggesting ways in which treatment might be made more culturally sensitive; (4) Addressing service delivery issues including the unique barriers Latino elders are likely to encounter and the impact of managed care; and (5) Advocating for increased resources for research and training to ameliorate the tremendous gaps in our knowledge base. In fact, if there is one theme that runs throughout this chapter it is the need for more systematically gathered information if the upcoming challenges are to be met.

Barbara Lynn Kail is Associate Professor, Fordham University Graduate School of Social Service. Mario DeLaRosa is Visiting Associate Research Professor, Boston University School of Social Work.

[Haworth co-indexing entry note]: "Challenges to Treating the Elderly Latino Substance Abuser: A Not So Hidden Research Agenda." Kail, Barbara Lynn, and Mario DeLaRosa. Co-published simultaneously in *Journal of Gerontological Social Work* (The Haworth Press, Inc.) Vol. 30, No. 1/2, 1998, pp. 123-141; and: *Latino Elders and the Twenty-First Century: Issues and Challenges for Culturally Competent Research and Practice* (ed: Melvin Delgado) The Haworth Press, Inc., 1998, pp. 123-141. Single or multiple copies of this article are available for a fee from The Haworth Document Delivery Service [1-800-342-9678, 9:00 a.m. - 5:00 p.m. (EST). E-mail address: getinfo@haworthpressinc.com].

© 1998 by The Haworth Press, Inc. All rights reserved.

THE EXTENT AND NATURE OF THE PROBLEM

Prevalence and Patterns of Drug Use

National data on the lifetime, past year, or past month prevalence of alcohol and other psychoactive drug use (e.g., benzodiazepams, marijuana, cocaine, heroin) among the Latino elderly are not available. The data available from the current National Household Survey on Drug Abuse (NHSDA), only report information on the prevalence of drug use among Latinos 35 years of age and older. These data may include some individuals over the age of 60 but do not report on them separately (Substance Abuse and Mental Health Administration, 1994). Data available from the NHSDA suggest that the use of alcohol, marijuana and cocaine drops off dramatically among Latinos as well as among other ethnic/racial groups when individuals are age 35 or older. However, this decrease in prevalence may conceal the fact that there is a smaller group who begin use and continue use into old age with continued problems, or that the problems do not persist after use ceases. (Substance Abuse and Mental Health Administration, 1994). NHSDA data also indicate that heavy alcohol and marijuana use was higher among individuals 35 years and older of Mexican ancestry than individuals from other Latino subgroups. Cocaine use was higher among individuals 35 years of age and older of Puerto Rican ancestry than individuals from other Latino groups. Finally, data from the 1993 NHSDA also indicate that alcohol use, including heavy alcohol use and other drug use, was higher among Latino males aged 35 and older than among Latino females aged 35 and older.

Data from earlier studies of Latino elderly drug behaviors seem to corroborate the 1993 NHSDA results. Caetano's study of Latino alcohol use patterns (1985) reports that alcohol use decreases with age. Further, Caetano (1985) found that among Latino men and women the rate of abstention remains stable until age 50-59 at which time it increases. Caetano (1985) also found that heavy alcohol use does persist into middle age among men and women. Among women, Caetano found that there is a group in their fifties that actually increases their alcohol use.

There are several patterns within these data worth noting. Similar to the NHSDA survey, Alcocer (1993) found that Latino men of all ages use alcohol more than Latino women. Alcocer (1993) also found that alcohol use by Latino elderly seems to indicate that they bring a pattern of infrequent but heavy consumption with them. In addition, data from a survey on the drug use behavior of Latino women found that Hispanic women over sixty reported higher rates and longer periods of Valium, Librium and Tranxene use than non-Latino women in this age group (Center for Substance Abuse Treatment, 1994).

Etiology of Drug Use

Systematic study of the underlying familial, community and societal factors responsible for the onset of substance abuse among the Latino elderly is not available. Research is needed which would explore whether the factors which have been found to be associated with the onset of alcohol and other drug use among Latino youth and young adults are similar to those found among elderly Latinos with early onset of alcohol and other drug use. Recent drug abuse research on Latino youth suggests that early onset of substance abuse among Latino youth is related to the stress associated with adjustment to American society and values (Vega et al., 1993). Other research on Latino youth has suggested that youth who receive strong support from their families were less likely to use drugs than Latino youth who receive no support from their families. This research also found that Latino youth who live in communities with low tolerance for drug use/dealing were less likely to use drugs than Latino youth who live in communities where drugs were readily available (Brook, 1993).

Similarly, there is no research on the etiology of "late onset" substance abuse among Latino elderly. Late onset appears to be a response to depression, bereavement, retirement, marital stress and illness (Zimber, 1985). Those with late onset report depression more frequently prior to their first drink. Rogler, Malgady and Rodriguez (1989) conclude from the available epidemiological literature that Latinos certainly present a profile of demographic characteristics that are associated with increased risk of mental disorder. Late onset is currently more likely to occur among women than men in the general population (Liberto & Oslin, 1997).

Additional research is also needed to determine the underlying factors responsible for gender differences in the patterns of use among Latinos of all ages. Past etiological research suggests that the higher incidence of early onset abuse among males may be related to Latino cultural values related to a particularly sharp demarcation of gender roles. These have been discussed extensively, often under the rubric of "machismo" (e.g., Bastida, 1988; Marin & Marin, 1991). Latino males have traditionally had more freedom to be in the "streets" and experiment with the use of alcohol and tobacco (Sanchez-Ayendez, 1988). However, other more recent studies suggest that as young Latina women acculturate into American society, the influences of the Latino culture and their families on drinking and other drug use lessens (Vega et al., 1993; Brook, 1993). Both U.S. born Latina adolescents and foreign born Latina adolescents who have acculturated to American values have drinking patterns similar to their male counterparts.

Summary

The limited information synthesized above suggests that substance abuse seems to be a less serious problem among Latino elderly than among Latino youth. The available data suggest that among Latino men who are heavy alcohol users, use persists into middle and old age. There are also data that suggest that Latina women of all ages are using alcohol and psychoactive substances with increasing frequency. In addition, our synthesis of available data also suggests that there is a cohort of Latina women age 60 and older who begin the use of alcohol and psychoactive drugs at this later point in their lives.

Clearly, one of the first challenges is the need for epidemiological studies that will address the incidence and prevalence of substance abuse among the Latino elderly. Samples of large national studies such as the NHSDA and Epidemiological Catchment Area studies need to be drawn in such a way that this subgroup is represented in sufficient numbers for analysis. Studies of Latino subgroups must include sufficient numbers of elders to make intracultural analysis possible. Finally, studies reassessing patterns of use, especially in light of acculturation and the aging of the baby boom generation, are essential to our understanding of the extent of this problem.

Other etiological research needs to explore whether there are different pathways to the development of drug using and misusing behaviors among early and late onset users. To what extent does the withdrawal of factors such as community and familial support and lack of access to drugs predict the "maturing out" of the early onset users–and how do these factors differ within the Latino community? How does acculturation and immigration affect both early and late onset among Latinos? These are just a few of the questions that might be posed.

IDENTIFICATION AND ASSESSMENT

The first task in treating older Latinos who abuse alcohol or other psychoactive substances is the identification and assessment of these individuals. In both areas, providers can expect to encounter challenges in the coming century.

Identification and Outreach

The elderly Latino who has aged into his substance use is likely to have come to the attention of gatekeepers to treatment through legal, financial and employment problems. (e.g., Liberto & Oslin, 1997) He may have a long history of being known to "the authorities" and may have experienced numerous rounds of prior detoxification and treatment that were unsuccessful.

The older Latina who begins substance abuse at a later age is much more difficult to reach out to and identify because of the synergistic effect of several values embedded in the Latino culture. The stigma attached to substance abuse by women within the larger culture (e.g., Ettore, 1992, Kendall, 1996) is probably heightened by the sharply demarcated gender role expectations within the Latino culture (Delgado & Humm-Delgado, 1993; DeLaRosa, 1990). These gender role expectations also make it less likely that substance abuse problems will come to the attention of others. For the elderly Latina, daily activities are centered around the home (Sanchez-Ayendez, 1988), and both drinking and taking medicines would probably be done in this setting, not in public (Gilbert, 1993; Delgado & Humm-Delgado, 1993).

The widely shared cultural value of "familismo" (Cervantes, 1993; Marin & Marin, 1991; Sanchez-Ayendez, 1988; Sotomayor & Applewhite, 1988) may translate into an approach that enables or hides grandma's alcohol or drug use. There are strong expectations that families will be the first and often only place one turns to in time of distress. Problems are to be kept within the family which is expected to deal with them as best as possible, especially since "washing dirty laundry in public" would embarrass the user and family.

The Latino value of respect for the elderly may reinforce the above value of "familismo" and prevent family members from discussing an older member's alcohol or other drug use (e.g., Sanchez-Ayendez, 1988). To do so could tarnish the image of the older individual and his/her family in the community.

If this particularly hidden population is to be reached, awareness of the problem must be heightened within several different systems. A first logical step is to sensitize providers of medical and substance abuse services within the Latino community. The traditionally received wisdom, extrapolated from the larger community of treatment providers and researchers, is that Latino substance abusers "mature out" of this behavior (e.g., Liberto & Oslin, 1997; Rosenberg, 1997; DesJarlais, Joseph & Courtwright, 1985; Glantz, 1985; Winick, 1962). These providers then do not expect to find older individuals in need of alcohol or drug abuse (AOD) treatment.

Efforts to raise awareness of those who provide a broad array of social services to the elderly, such as senior citizen recreational activities and meals on wheels, might also prove very useful in reaching out and identifying those at risk. Social workers may be another target for educational efforts given this profession's tradition of holistic assessment and ties to a number of different services (Raffoul & Haney, 1993). Social workers may also be key in invoking the informal social networks, identifying leaders within the community and drawing on community organization skills to heighten awareness.

The informal social support systems within Latino communities are key to identifying and reaching out to the older Latino substance abuser. These informal systems have successfully provided an array of social and economic assistance to the Latino elderly. This network of informal support could be rallied to make the community aware of the problem of substance abuse among the Latino elderly (Delgado & Humm-Delgado, 1982; DeLaRosa, 1988). These informal support systems are also unique in their ability to address the values that act as barriers, possibly paving the way for a greater acceptance that such problems do indeed exist and are not cause for shame.

Assessment

Once identified, the elderly Latino who abuses alcohol or psychoactive substances must be assessed. We anticipate that in the twenty-first century, providers will be increasingly asked to show that they can screen effectively for the appropriate level of substance abuse treatment and assess the outcomes of that treatment. This makes the development of culturally sensitive techniques for the Latino elderly all the more important. Currently existing instruments are less than optimal or at times inappropriate for use with the Latino elderly. They suffer from a number of problems including measurement validity; potentially poor reliability; communication problems including translation issues; administration by poorly trained gatekeepers.

The development or adaptation of existing substance abuse assessment instruments for Latino elderly needs to address the following dimensions: physiological symptoms of dependence on alcohol or other drugs, pathological use of alcohol or other drugs and social impairment associated with drug use. These three dimensions have been found to be critical in accurately and validly assessing whether a person is experiencing a substance abuse problem and the severity of their problem (DeHart & Hoffman, 1997).

Physiological symptoms of abuse such as confusion and dementia, difficulty sleeping, and gastrointestinal distress mimic some of the normal processes of aging, making it difficult to determine the extent of the problem among Latino elderly. These symptoms may be compounded by the stress associated with adjustment to the larger Anglo society and attempts at acculturation that the elderly Latino is likely to experience (Rogler, Malgady & Rodriguez, 1989). Therefore, some of these physiological measures of substance dependency may be inappropriate for this population.

Assessing pathological use of alcohol or drugs presents other measurement difficulties. Traditionally this aspect of assessment has centered around: continued use despite recurrent physical or psychological problems; scheduling one's day to accommodate use; and the amount of time spent acquiring, using and recovering from use. Some of these criteria need to be rethought for the elderly Latino. For the older Latina dependent on Valium, this may mean inquiring about trips to the doctors office, submitting to medical tests, trips to the pharmacy, calls for refills, and asking for assistance in all these activities, especially where translation is needed. Other aspects of pathological use may need to be rethought as well.

Finally, measures of social impairment included in these assessments are often inappropriate to the Latino elderly and need to be reconsidered when used to assess the Latino elderly. Grahm (1986) notes that the problems currently used as markers of alcoholism and drug use have been standardized on young males–physical aggression, driving while intoxicated, legal problems, employment problems. A retired elderly Latino male or an elderly Latina is not likely to have employment obligations, and may not own or drive a car. The family obligations measured should be culturally sensitive to the expectations that Latino elderly provide: assistance with child care and discipline; emotional support and advice especially in times of crisis; and socialization across generations into the cultural values of the family (Sotomayor & Applewhite, 1988). Measures of social impairment could include problems in meeting the responsibilities just outlined. One might also add to the list an increase in complaints of illnesses traditionally treated by curanderos (faith healers) or increased use of home remedies to self medicate and trips to the botanica. We have not even touched on the notion that some of the home remedies and teas bought at the botanica, and prescribed by herbalists, may have psychoactive properties that could be abused.

The reliability of existing assessment instruments for the Latino elderly may also be problematic. Almost without exception, assessment instruments include a series of simple questions about frequency and amount of use. Such questions are particularly problematic for the Latino elderly. Self reports require an accurate memory, which in the Latino elderly may be impaired by both cognitive losses and the substance use itself (Grahm, 1986). Furthermore, the elderly (Grahm, 1986), and especially the Latino elderly, both male and particularly female, may be prone to deny or minimize their use because of the cultural values described above.

The training of gatekeepers in the use of any instruments developed is essential. There are indications that both issues of communication and differences in expectations of the encounter may impede understanding between the elderly Latino client and assessor (Garrity & Lawson, 1989). The individual making the assessment may not be Latino. Even if the individual is Latino, there is no guarantee that simple cultural concordance will bridge socio-economic and intracultural differences (Facundo, 1991).

Finally, at its most basic, there is the issue of language, crucial for a population that can be expected to be largely Spanish-speaking (Trevino, 1988). Assessment instruments must be available in both Spanish and English. To ensure comparability, they should be translated from English to Spanish and back-translated into English. Instruments should also be reviewed to insure that meanings of particular words are not local to one geographic area (Marin & Marin, 1991).

Summary

Finding and assessing the elderly Latino who abuses alcohol or psychoactive substances presents unique challenges. The Latina who begins use at an older age may be particularly difficult to identify. She and her family may both be inclined to deny the problem. Providers of both social services to the elderly and alcohol and other drug treatment may also not be attuned to this problem, relying on the received wisdom that these problems are of the young, and abusers either die or "mature out." Testing the impact of educating gatekeepers within the community would advance our knowledge in this area. Further research on how the informal support system might be educated to recognize this problem could also substantially add to our knowledge base, as might efforts to address some of the culturally-based barriers discussed above.

Instruments used to assess the Latino elderly for such problems present issues of applicability of content and reliability of responses. Traditional measures of physiological symptoms of dependence and social impairment may be inappropriate for elderly Latinos. Even simple questions of amount and frequency, included in all assessment instruments, will suffer from problems of communication, exacerbated by denial and cognitive impairment. Once created, there remain issues of translation and training of gatekeepers.

Although some empirical work has been done in the area of screening and outcome measures for the elderly, the applicability of existing measures such as the MAST-G and the Drinking Problem Index (DeHarte & Hoffman, 1997) to a Latino population is unclear. Perhaps the initial research in this important area might be translating and validating these instruments on a Spanish-speaking population, Further work to determine appropriate indicators of substance abuse, especially in the area of social impairment among the Latino elderly, could improve the validity of these instruments.

TREATMENT

The twenty-first century can be expected to bring at least two treatment issues that must be addressed if the elderly Latino substance abuser is to be well served. The first is the development of placement criteria appropriate to this sub-population. With managed care and the drive to treat in the least restrictive setting, such criteria can only gain in importance. The second issue is that of modifying existing treatment to be culturally sensitive to the needs of the Latino elderly.

Placement Criteria

We anticipate the coming century will bring increasing calls for standardized placement criteria in an effort to both increase the appropriateness of treatment and contain costs. This can be expected to result in a certain amount of tension in attempting to apply such criteria to minority populations in treatment–and the Latino elderly are indeed a double minority. Perhaps the most widely used criteria are the American Society for Addiction Medicine (ASAM) Criteria. These criteria include six dimensions of assessment: acute intoxication; biomedical complications; emotional/behavioral complications; treatment acceptance/resistance; relapse potential; and recovery environment. These dimensions require modification for the Latino elderly if they are not to result in an automatic placement in a more restrictive level of care than might be warranted. Their emotional and behavioral complications are likely to be different, including higher levels of stigma and shame as mentioned in the section on outreach. Their resistance to treatment is also likely to be higher given cultural beliefs that alcohol or drug use may be the result of moral failings (Delgado & Humm-Delgado, 1993) or connected to mental illness, which is also stigmatized (e.g., Rogler Malgady & Rodriguez, 1989). Assessment of the recovery environment needs to include an assessment of the family and the role the elderly individual plays. For Latino elderly this may also mean casting a wider net, including ties to extended family and friends brought into the family through compadrazgo.

Modifications to Existing Treatment Modalities

We found no literature on substance abuse treatment for the Latino elderly. In reviewing the small body of alcohol or drug (AOD) treatment for the elderly and the equally small body of literature on AOD treatment for Latinos, we suggest that providers might make some of the following changes to enhance the cultural sensitivity of their treatment. We do wish to note that prior to even considering modifications for treatment, it is essential that providers be bilingual. The elderly are not likely to participate, especially those less acculturated, unless they are comfortable in the language. Applewhite and Daley (1988) report that the availability of bilingual/bicultural therapists is an important influence on the utilization of social services. Pinsker (1985) anecdotally reports an inability to involve his Latino clients in English-speaking groups.

It may be helpful to slow the pace of treatment for Latino elderly clients. Several authors note that for the elderly, the pace of counseling, group therapy and educational programs must be slower because of the cognitive and sensory losses that often accompany aging (Finlayson, 1997; Schoenfeld & Dupree, 1997) It may be unwise to use fast paced films and curriculum developed to meet the needs of younger substance abusers. Issues of simplicity and pace become even more salient for the Latino elderly given potential barriers to understanding posed by differences between provider and client in language, social class and expectations. Finlayson (1997) suggests that, in general, the elderly will retain information better if they are provided with some individual instruction that repeats the information provided in group sessions. Garrity and Lawson (1989) echo this advice for the Latino client, suggesting repetition, simplicity of sentences, specificity of advice and the arrangement of advice in categories.

The content of the curriculum in traditional psychosocial and cognitive therapeutic models could also be modified to be more culturally sensitive to the needs of the Latino elderly. Groups may be used to address issues of loss, depression and isolation brought on by aging and immigration. (Schoefeld & Dupree, 1997). Issues of acculturation and differences in expectations among generations may become particularly salient.

Involvement of the family, especially for those late onset clients who have retained ties, should be culturally sensitive. The older Latina may be more likely than her Anglo or African-American counterparts to retain the support of her family, and ties to grown children and extended family may remain strong. Sotomayor and Applewhite (1988) describe the Latino elderly as embedded in a social network based on kin or kin-type relationships. However, several values–"familismo," "respeto" and the stigma associated with violation of clearly demarcated gender expectations may result in the family's closing its eyes to grandma's problem and possibly enabling her (e.g., Marin & Marin, 1991; Paz & Applewhite, 1988; Sanchez-Ayendez, 1988).

The use of confrontation, often associated with therapeutic communities and Alcoholics Anonymous, may be less tolerated by the elderly Latino client. The Latino client is likely to carry expectations that social interactions be conducted in a manner characterized by "respeto" and "simpatia." The value of "simpatia" places a premium on graciousness, harmony and the avoidance of conflict (Delgado & Humm-Delgado, 1993; Marin & Marin, 1991). The values of "respeto and "dignidad" imply that power differentials between individuals are understood, but that individuals are to feel that their own personal power, whatever it may be, is acknowledged–they should be allowed to retain some "face." To these expectations, the elderly bring further expectations of "respeto" and "dignidad" based on age. Both Sanchez-Ayendez (1988) and Paz and Applewhite (1988) note that within the Latino culture the elderly are accorded substantial status and respect, with positive cultural norms around aging in opposition to the ageism likely to be found in the larger society. Confrontational techniques appear to be almost diametrically opposed to the culturally-based expectations outlined above.

There is one last issue in the treatment of alcohol and drug abuse that is particular to the treatment of Latinos: the role of acculturation. We may increasingly find two very different groups of elderly among the Latino population–an extremely acculturated group who aged while living in the U.S. and another group of recent immigrants who are less acculturated. The experiences and values these two groups bring to treatment are likely to be quite different.

Summary

The existing literature on substance abuse treatment of elderly Latinos suggests that several modifications be made. To begin, it is important that the services be offered by bi-lingual workers who have the ability to tailor the language to the preferences of their clients. The material we have synthesized also suggests that a slower pace and content that is sensitive to the particular issues of the Latino elderly be utilized. Work with the families of elderly Latino clients should be sensitive to the value of "familismo," drawing on its strengths to involve available family–nuclear, extended and adopted–and minimizing their tendency to withdraw into themselves in times of difficulties. The use of confrontation, so typical of certain AOD treatment modalities, seems to be particularly inappropriate for the older Latino. Acculturation, and in particular the possibility that providers could be treating Latino elderly of widely varying levels of acculturation, should color the use of the above suggestions.

Having said all of the above, we are left with the astounding fact that little if any of these suggestions are based on a firm knowledge that when implemented they will be effective. Our efforts at reviewing the literature yielded only anecdotal documentation of substance abuse treatment that could be applied to our sub-population. We recommend that researchers begin here, evaluating existing programs in Latino communities. From there, further studies might look at the impact of some of the modifications we recommended above and their relative effect on outcomes. Contrasting different modalities and their effectiveness would refine our knowledge.

SERVICE DELIVERY ISSUES

The delivery of services to the elderly Latino who has a substance abuse problem may face two challenges in the coming century. One is the extent to which services should be specialized and their placement within the delivery system. The second is the impact of managed care as a means of delivery.

Specialization of Services

Providers of substance abuse treatment to the Latino elderly will not find a clear-cut message in the literature as to the extent of specialization needed. Some authors argue that until research indicates that age-specific substance abuse treatment is more effective than age-heterogeneous models, there is no reason to separate the elderly out; the main problem is the addiction which overrides all other issues (Mishara, 1985; Pinsker, 1985; Solomon, Manepallim, Ireland & Mahon, 1993). Others suggest that the problems of the elderly are so unique–and by inference those of the Latino elderly are even more so–that services must be age-homogeneous (Finlayson, 1997; Mishara, 1985; Schoenfeld & Dupree, 1997; Zimber, 1985). We suggest that the argument is not nearly so simple. The "drug culture" of the individual, reflected by gender and age of onset, may determine the need for treatment in age-homogeneous groups.

Latino men coming to treatment with a long history of substance abuse and prior treatment experience are much more likely to resemble their younger counterparts. They may have had a great deal of experience with prior attempts at treatment and be comfortable in the traditional treatment setting. Some specialized programming is certainly called for, but might well be handled within the setting. One provider reported anecdotally that group sessions of older Latino men in a traditional treatment setting did not address issues of aging but tended to include a certain amount of mirthful boasting and talk of women (Pinsker, 1985).

Older Latina women who begin use at an older age present a different set of treatment needs. Older Latina women adhere to very clear norms concerning what is permissible to discuss outside the family, particularly concerning sex (Bastida, 1988). They would be extremely uncomfortable within the treatment environment described above. Their issues around loss, separation and acculturation are also likely to be gender-determined.

It may be particularly important, then, to treat the Latino elderly in groups based on gender and onset, which may well overlap. Delgado and Humm-Delgado (1993) echo this recommendation, suggesting that self-help groups such as Alcoholics Anonymous be organized along gender lines for Latinos.

Yet a second issue is that of where these services should be placed: within a specialized drug and alcohol setting, a mental health setting or a medical setting. Arguments could be made for the virtues of each. The specialized substance abuse provider has expertise with existing modalities and may be very familiar and acceptable to early onset users. There are at least two studies of older heroin users who find methadone maintenance programs to be a haven when reliable sources of the drug begin to fail (DeJarlais et al., 1985; Rosenblatt, 1997). The Latino who ages into his drug or alcohol use may react similarly. On the other hand, location within a mental health or medical setting may be somewhat more acceptable to the late onset user, given the stigma attached to substance abuse (Delgado & Humm-Delgado, 1993). The Latino elderly and their families may be more willing to consider the problem one of "nervios" or anxiety, suggesting a mental health setting.

However, we do wish to note that mental health services carry with them their own set of assumptions and stigma within the Latino community (Delgado & Humm-Delgado, 1993; Rogler; Malgady & Rodriguez, 1989). A medical setting may be most acceptable to the Latina late onset user and appropriate given the greater likelihood of medical complications among this group simply due to age and the potential number of other medications and drug interactions.

The Impact of Managed Care

Managed care may well shape how services will be delivered in the twenty-first century. The current model typically offers services through a Health Maintenance Organization, paid on a capitation rather than fee-for-service basis. Delivery is presumably characterized by greater emphasis on prevention to avoid more costly treatment and by gatekeeping mechanisms to avoid unnecessary and duplicative services. To the extent that elderly Latino Medicare and Medicaid recipients are enrolled in Health Maintenance Organizations they will be particularly affected.

Delivery through an HMO mechanism could decrease the likelihood of identifying older Latino substance abusers. Payment on a capitation basis means there is less incentive to identify a population that is costly and resistant to treatment. HMOs must be convinced that it is in their interest to identify the elderly Latino abuser to forestall some of the other expensive medical complications that may arise. HMOs tend to lack ties to community-based organizations that might assist in the identification of Latino elderly having difficulties (CSAT 1995a; CSAT 1995b). However, the increasing use of gatekeepers within medical settings who might be trained may make identification and referral easier.

Once identified, delivery through an HMO may facilitate or hinder successful engagement of the Latino elderly. The Latino elderly may find that the plan they have enrolled in covers only a limited amount of coverage for alcohol and drug treatment, insufficient for early onset users who may require many courses of treatment. Late onset Latina users may be unable to find specialized services within their plan. Including "any willing provider" clauses in State contracts with HMOs may help alleviate some of these problems, allowing for a greater range of community based organizations to compete for specialized service contracts with the HMO.

The consumer protections provided by the HMO are particularly important to the elderly Latino substance abuser and should be reviewed by state agencies contracting with HMOs. Criteria for placement should be clear and easily available to the consumer for an open discussion of cultural issues. Consumer friendly materials concerning available benefits and appeal processes in clearly written Spanish should be distributed by providers. Disenrollment protections should be in place so that when identified, the elderly Latino substance abuser is not "dumped." The availability of out of plan services could be particularly important to older Latinos who might find only one or two local providers of services that meet their needs.

Summary

The extent of specialization and location of these specialized services would seem to differ a bit for late and early onset users. We suggest early onset Latino users socialized into a more youthful drug and alcohol culture may require somewhat less specialized services. This is not to say that they can be well served without differentiation from their younger counterparts, but that specialized groups or other services such as linkages with medical settings and possibly nursing homes may be sufficient. Older Latinas who begin substance abuse at a later age present a very different picture and are likely to require very specialized services if they are to be engaged and their treatment issues addressed. These highly specialized services might be better delivered within a medical setting as opposed to substance abuse or mental health settings.

Managed care and delivery through HMOs may restrict access and services but has the potential to increasingly engage the Latino elderly. There is currently little incentive for outreach and identification. However, the use of gatekeepers, along with a more preventive orientation, could result in more extensive training of primary care physicians to recognize the problem. The particular HMO an elderly Latino is enrolled in may not cover the amount of service needed or the specialized service. However, inclusion of a greater range of community based services and provisions for out of plan coverage may help alleviate this problem. Finally, the Latino elderly will be in particular need of consumer protection.

We wish again to highlight the paucity of empirical data in this area. The information synthesized above is largely based on anecdotal description and theoretical pieces. We suggest that one area of fruitful research might center around the types of settings most amenable to these services. To what extent do elderly Latinos find particular settings more or less acceptable? Does this differ by gender and onset? What is the reaction of their families to different settings? Yet another set of research issues comes with the increasing implementation of managed care and delivery through HMOs. An economic analysis of the costs of untreated substance abuse among the Latino elderly would add great depth to our knowledge base and perhaps have the added impact of increasing the incentive for outreach. The impact of gatekeeping mechanisms, financing and coverage as barriers is also a ripe area for investigation. Finally, we have yet to speak of the "indocumentados," those here without legal papers. We suspect that if they receive services at all, it is only through acute care in emergency rooms; at what cost to them and society?

RESEARCH FUNDING AND TRAINING ISSUES

It seems only logical to us then that we end our chapter with a call for both funding and trained investigators who can address the research agenda proposed throughout this chapter.

Research Funding Issues

Funding organizations need to increase the funding levels for research on the drug-using behavior of Latino elderly and the effectiveness of drug treatment programs to address the drug problem among Latino elderly. Program announcements requesting drug abuse researchers to submit for funding for research projects focusing on Latino elderly drug behaviors could be used by funding organizations to spur interest in this area of research. Further, there is a need for funding organizations to conduct research conferences to assess the state of knowledge in research on Latino elderly. The results from these conferences could be utilized to develop a future research agenda for the conduct of drug abuse research on Latino elderly.

Training Students

Academic programs need to train students to become researchers in conducting drug abuse with Latino elderly populations. Programs to train students need to be developed or expanded to provide substantive information on culture, community and minority status factors affecting the drug behaviors of Latino elderly. As part of this expansion, they need to teach students how to measure these factors in Latino elderly populations. In addition, programs need to encourage students to expand their knowledge of constructs from other disciplines which are relevant to the study of drug behaviors in Latino elderly. Finally, programs need to teach students ethnographic and other methods which have been found to be effective in collecting data from hard-to-reach populations such as the Latino elderly.

CONCLUSION

We can only emphasize that in the twenty-first century the treatment of older Latino substance abusers will increasingly become an issue. As discussed in other chapters contained in this volume, the numbers of Hispanics living in this country are increasing. Some are becoming older, having spent their lives in the U.S.; others arrive at an older age. Added to these increasing numbers are several phenomenon that can be expected to increase the extent of substance abuse and associated problems: increasing numbers of Hispanics who begin using drugs and alcohol when young who may be expected to age; an increasingly tolerant attitude toward the use of psychoactive substances by acculturated Latinos belonging to the baby boom generation; and increasing access to medical care and prescribed medications compared to earlier generations. We can no longer close our eyes to the dearth of information on how to reach out, assess, treat and deliver services to this population

REFERENCES

Alcocer, A. (1993). Patterns of alcohol use among Hispanics. In Mayers, R.S., Kail, B. & Watts, T. (Eds.), *Hispanic Substance Abuse.* (pp. 37-50). Springfield, IL: Charles C Thomas Publishers

Aleman, S. (1997) *Hispanic elders and human services.* New York: Garland Publishing.

Applewhite, S. & Daley, J. (1988). Cross cultural understanding for social work practice with the Hispanic elderly. In S. R. Applewhite (Ed.), *Hispanic elderly in transition: Theory, research, policy and practice* (pp. 1-17). Westport CT: Greenwood Press.

Bastida, E. (1988). Age and gender linked norms among older Hispanic women. In S. R. Applewhite (Ed.), *Hispanic elderly in transition: Theory research policy and practice* (pp. 159-170). Westport CT: Greenwood Press.

Brook, J. (1993). Interactional Theory: Its utility in explaining drug use behavior among African-American and Puerto Rican youth. In M.R. DeLaRosa & J Recio-Adrados (Eds.), *Drug abuse among minority youth: Advances in research and methodology* (pp. 79-101). *National Institute on Drug Abuse Research Monograph 130* (NIH Publication No. 93-3479). Washington DC: U.S. Department of Health and Human Services.

Caetano, R. (1985, September). *Drinking patterns and alcohol problems in a national sample of U.S. Hispanics.* Paper presented at the National Institute of Alcohol Abuse and Alcoholism Conference, Epidemiology of Alcohol Use and Abuse Among U.S. Minorities, Bethesda, MD.

Cervantes, R. (1993). The Hispanic family intervention program: An empirical approach to substance abuse prevention. In Mayers, R.S., Kail, B. & Watts, T. (Eds.), *Hispanic Substance Abuse* (pp. 101-114). Springfield, IL: Charles C Thomas Publishers.

Center for Substance Abuse Treatment (CSAT) (1994). *Practical approaches in the treatment of women who abuse alcohol and other drugs.* (DHHS Publication No SMA 94-3006). Washington DC: U.S. Government Printing Office.

Center for Substance Abuse Treatment (CSAT) (1995a). *Purchasing managed care services for alcohol and other drug treatment* (DHHS Publication No. SMA 96-3091). Washington DC: U.S. Government Printing Office.

Center for Substance Abuse Treatment (CSAT) (1995b). Managed care: meeting the challenge to substance abuse treatment. *Treatment Improvement Exchange Communique, Spring.* Washington, DC: U.S.Government Printing Office.

DeHart, S. & Hoffman, N.G. (1997). Screening and Diagnosis: alcohol use disorders in older adults. In Gurnack, A.M. (Ed.), *Older adult's misuse of alcohol, medicines and other drugs* (pp. 25-53). New York: Springer Publishing Co.

DeLaRosa, M.R. (1988). Natural support systems of Hispanics: A key dimension for their well-being. *Health and Social Work, 15,* 181-190.

DeLaRosa, M.R., Khalsa, J.H. & Rouse, B.A. (1990). Hispanics and illicit drug use: A review of recent findings. *The International Journal of the Addictions, 25,* 665-691.

Delgado, M. & Humm-Delgado, D. (1982). Natural support systems: Sources of strength in Hispanic communities. *Social Work, 27,* 83-89.

Delgado, M. & Humm-Delgado, D. (1993). Chemical dependence, self help groups and the Hispanic community. In Mayers, R.S., Kail, B. & Watts, T. (Eds.), *Hispanic Substance Abuse* (pp. 145-156). Springfield, IL: Charles C Thomas Publishers.

Des Jarlais, D., Joseph H. & Courtwright W. (1985). Old age and addiction: a study of elderly patients in methadone maintenance treatment. In E. Gottheil, K. A. Druly, T.E. Skoloda & H.M. Waxman (Eds.), *The combined problems of alcoholism, drug addiction and aging* (pp. 201-208). Springfield, IL: Charles C Thomas Publishers.

Ettore, E. (1992). *Women and substance abuse.* New Jersey: Rutgers University Press.

Facundo, A. (1991). Sensitive mental health services for low-income Puerto Rican Families. In M. Sotomayor (Ed.), *Empowering Hispanic families: A critical issue for the '90s.* (pp. 121-140). Milwaukee, WI: Family Service America.

Finlayson, R. (1997). Misuse of prescription drugs. In Gurnack, A.M. (Ed.), *Older adult's misuse of alcohol, medicines and other drugs* (pp. 158-184). New York: Springer Publishing Co.

Garrity & Lawson (1989). Patient physician communication as a determinant of medication misuse in older, minority women. *Journal of Drug Issues, 19,* 245-260.

Gilbert, J. (1993). Intracultural variation in alcohol-related cognitions among Mexican-Americans. In Mayers, R.S., Kail, B. & Watts, T. (Eds.), *Hispanic Substance Abuse.* (pp. 51-64). Springfield, IL: Charles C Thomas Publishers.

Gilbert, J. & Cervantes, R. (1986). Patterns and practices of alcohol use among Mexican Americans: A comprehensive review. *Hispanic Journal of Behavioral Sciences, 8,* 1-60.

German, P. & Burton, L.C. (1989). Clinicians, the elderly and drugs. *Journal of Drug Issues, 19(2),* 221-243.

Glantz, M. (1985). The detection, identification and differentiation of elderly drug misuse and abuse in a research survey. In E. Gottheil, K. A. Druly, T.E. Skoloda &

H.M. Waxman (Eds.), *The combined problems of alcoholism, drug addiction and aging* (pp. 113-129). Springfield, IL: Charles C Thomas Publishers.

Grahm, K. (1986). Identifying and measuring alcohol abuse among the elderly: Serious problems with existing instrumentation. *Journal of Studies on Alcohol, 47,* 322-326.

Kendall, S. (1996). *Substance and shadow: Women and addiction in the US.* Cambridge: Harvard University Press.

Liberto, J. & Oslin, D.W. (1997). Early versus late onset of alcoholism in the elderly. In Gurnack, A.M. (Ed.), *Older adult's misuse of alcohol, medicines and other drugs* (pp. 94-112). New York: Springer Publishing Co.

Marin, G. & Marin, B. Van Oss (1991). *Research with Hispanic populations.* Newbury Park CA: Sage Publications.

Mishara, B. (1985). What we know, don't know and need to know about older alcoholics and how to help them: models of prevention and treatment. In E. Gottheil, K. A. Druly, T.E. Skoloda & H.M. Waxman (Eds.), *The combined problems of alcoholism, drug addiction and aging* (pp. 243-261). Springfield, IL: Charles C Thomas Publishers.

Pinsker, H. (1985). Outpatient treatment of older alcoholics. In E. Gottheil, K. A. Druly, T.E. Skoloda & H.M. Waxman (Eds.), *The combined problems of alcoholism, drug addiction and aging* (pp. 278-283). Springfield, IL: Charles C Thomas Publishers.

Paz, E. & Applewhite, S. (1988). Empowerment: Strengthening the natural support network of the Hispanic rural elderly. In S. R. Applewhite (Ed.), *Hispanic elderly in transition: Theory research policy and practice* (pp. 143-157). Westport CT: Greenwood Press.

Raffoul & Haney (1989). Interdisciplinary treatment of drug misuse among older people of color: Ethnic considerations for social work practice. *Journal of Drug Issues, 19,* 297-311.

Rogler, L., Rodriguz, O. & Malgady, R. (1989). *Hispanics and mental health: A framework for research.* Malabar FL: Krieger Publishing Co.

Rosenberg, H. (1997). Use and abuse of illicit drugs among older people. In Gurnack, A.M. (Ed.), *Older adult's misuse of alcohol, medicines and other drugs* (pp. 206-227). New York: Springer Publishing Co.

Sanchez-Ayendez, M. (1988). Elderly Puerto Ricans in the United States. In S. R. Applewhite (Ed.), *Hispanic elderly in transition: Theory, research, policy and practice* (pp. 17-32). Westport CT: Greenwood Press.

Schoenfeld, L. & Dupree, L. (1997). Treatment alternatives for older alcohol abusers. In Gurnack, A.M. (Ed.), *Older adult's misuse of alcohol, medicines and other drugs* (pp. 113-131). New York: Springer Publishing Co.

Solomon, K., Manepallim, J., Ireland, G.A. & Mahon, G.M. (1993). Alcholism and prescription drug abuse in the elderly: St. Louis University grand rounds. *American Geriatric Society, 41,* 57-69.

Sotomayor, M. & Applewhite, S. (1988). The Hispanic elderly and the extended multigenerational family. In S. R. Applewhite (Ed.), *Hispanic elderly in transition: Theory, research, policy and practice* (pp. 121-134). Westport CT: Greenwood Press.

Substance Abuse and Mental Health Services Administration. (1994). *National Household Survey on Drug Abuse: Population Estimates, October 1994* (DHHS Pub. No. ADM 94-3017). Washington DC: US Government Printing Office.

Trevino, M. (1988). A comparative analysis of need, access and utilization of health and human services. In S. R. Applewhite (Ed.), *Hispanic elderly in transition: Theory, research, policy and practice* (pp. 61-72). Westport CT: Greenwood Press.

Vega, W., Gil, A., Warheit, G., Zimmerman, R. & Apospori, E. (1993). Acculturation and delinquent behavior among Cuban adolescents: Toward an empirical model. *Journal of Community Psychology, 21*, pp. 113-125.

Winick, C. (1962). Maturing out of narcotic addiction. *Bulletin on Narcotics, 14*, 1-7.

Zimberg, S. (1985). Treatment of the elderly alcoholic. In E. Gottheil, K. A. Druly, T.E. Skoloda & H.M. Waxman (Eds.), *The combined problems of alcoholism, drug addiction and aging* (pp. 284-299). Springfield, IL: Charles C Thomas Publishers.

Social Policy
and the Politics of Hispanic Aging

Fernando M. Torres-Gil, PhD
TsuAnn Kuo, MSW

The passage of the 1996 Welfare Reform Bill highlighted the vulnerability of elderly immigrants in American politics. The elimination of public benefits to legal immigrants and the subsequent restoration of some of those benefits to older and disabled immigrants illustrates the tremendous stake that Hispanics and other minorities have in the electoral process and in political participation. Those political events, however, also give the impression that immigrants, particularly Hispanic elders, are a disenfranchised group beholden to advocates and sympathetic politicians on whom they depend to protect their interests. This article posits that the actual political participation of Hispanic elders may in fact suggest an emerging politics of aging in the Hispanic community, one that can influence social welfare and social policy.

Fernando M. Torres-Gil is Professor of Social Welfare and Policy Studies, and Director, Center for Policy Research on Aging, School of Public Policy and Social Research, University of California, Los Angeles (UCLA). TsuAnn Kuo is a doctoral student, Department of Social Welfare, and Research Assistant, Center for Policy Research on Aging, School of Public Policy and Social Research, UCLA.

Address correspondence to Fernando M. Torres-Gil, 3250 Public Policy Building, Box 951656, UCLA School of Public Policy and Social Research, Los Angeles, CA 90095-1656.

The authors extend appreciation to Valentine Villa, PhD, Lisa Nguyen, MSW, and Michelle Putnam, MGS, for their invaluable assistance, and acknowledge the support of the Center for Policy Research on Aging, UCLA School of Public Policy and Social Research.

[Haworth co-indexing entry note]: "Social Policy and the Politics of Hispanic Aging." Torres-Gil, Fernando M., and TsuAnn Kuo. Co-published simultaneously in *Journal of Gerontological Social Work* (The Haworth Press, Inc.) Vol. 30, No. 1/2, 1998, pp. 143-158; and: *Latino Elders and the Twenty-First Century: Issues and Challenges for Culturally Competent Research and Practice* (ed: Melvin Delgado) The Haworth Press, Inc., 1998, pp. 143-158. Single or multiple copies of this article are available for a fee from The Haworth Document Delivery Service [1-800-342-9678, 9:00 a.m. - 5:00 p.m. (EST). E-mail address: getinfo@haworthpressinc.com].

143

This article examines voting and other vehicles of political participation by Hispanic elders and raises implications for social policy and a politics of aging in the Hispanic community. While much has been written about the politics of aging and the role of older persons in public policy and the political process, a paucity of research exists about Hispanic elders as a potential political factor in social policy (Torres-Gil, 1982). In light of the fact that Hispanics and older persons are the two fastest growing interest groups in the United States, it is useful, and even necessary, to understand the myths and realities of political participation by older Hispanics.

THE POLITICS OF SOCIAL POLICY

Social policy is a product of politics and the political process. Ongoing debates about health care reform, entitlement changes and budgetary decisions affecting federal and state programs underscore the joint influence of interest group politics, political decisions and public opinion on the passage and implementation of social policies. Increasingly, policy decisions are also shaped by the ability of political constituencies to mobilize and influence political leaders and public opinion.

The passage of the Personal Responsibility and Work Opportunity Reconciliation Act of 1996 (welfare reform) and the portrayal of immigrants as an "undeserving" group exemplify the nature of interest group politics and the consequences of diminished political clout. As welfare reform proposals were debated in the Congress, the White House and the Department of Health and Human Services from 1993 through 1996, it became clear that there was ineffective mobilization by advocates for the poor, social service providers, welfare recipients and immigrants. The key players in influencing the final passage of this bill included state governors, Republican party officials, conservative organizations, and an elite media that portrayed these groups as undeserving, an economic drain, and in need of behavioral changes. Advocates such as the National Association of Social Welfare (NASW) and child welfare organizations did their best but were unable to overcome public antipathy toward the status quo and the fragmentation among these competing groups. The final bill eliminated the entitlement status of the Aid to Families with Dependent Children (AFDC) program, imposed time limits for the receipt of public benefits and instituted work-requirements. Some positive benefits did arise such as an expanded child care block grant and greater discretion for state and county governments to design social service programs.

Immigrant elders were especially hard hit when they were denied Supplemental Security Income (SSI) and food stamps; and states were given discretion to eliminate Medicaid and other state-funded benefits. Despite the best efforts of the Hispanic and Asian congressional caucuses, the Personal Responsibility and Work Opportunity Act of 1996 became law. This loss reflected congressional efforts to achieve budget savings (the largest savings came from eliminating immigrant benefits), as well as public ambivalence about high rates of immigration and insufficient lobbying and advocacy by advocates.

Fortunately, within a year of the bill's implementation, the Congress, through the Balanced Budget Act of 1997, restored some benefits to immigrants and the disabled–SSI for immigrants already enrolled and SSI disability to severely disabled children. The reasons for this reversal came largely from a sympathetic media portrayal of the dire consequences for elderly immigrants (e.g., loss of nursing home care), the realization by state governors with a high proportion of immigrants that they would lose federal dollars, and belated organizing by grassroots groups, welfare department directors and elected officials, including advocates for Armenians, Asians, Russian Jews and Hispanics.

The successful outcome of this case, however, does not detract from the central theme of this article–the need to define new political constituency groups that can bolster the influence of coalitions seeking to protect services and benefits. For example, legal immigrants–and elderly immigrants who do not become citizens–remain vulnerable and cannot afford to rely on public sympathy and supportive elected officials. California's proposition 187, which attempted to eliminate state services to immigrants, and Proposition 209, which banned the use of affirmative action programs based on race, as well as federal efforts to do the same (e.g., The Aderand Decision), place constant pressure on advocates and affected constituents to organize, mobilize and play the interest group game. On a macro level, bipartisan agreement to eliminate the deficit over the next five years and the concomitant downsizing of federal funds and agencies will bring increasing pressure on advocates to preserve and protect social services and benefits.

POLITICS OF AGING

In contrast to the difficulties that social welfare advocates faced with welfare reform, the passage and implementation of entitlement reform affecting older persons demonstrates the political influence and sophisticated mobilization of senior citizens. During the time that the Congress and the Executive branch were debating how best to "end welfare as we know it" and to achieve a bipartisan compromise on balancing the federal budget, programs for older persons were also threatened. Medicare, Medicaid and Social Security, which are the bedrock of social welfare for older persons and their families, embodying the last vestiges of the New Deal–the "social contract" that implicitly promised that the elderly would receive health and economic security in their old age–have been shaken. There have been proposals to means-test Part B (medical insurance) of the Medicare Program by imposing higher premiums on affluent beneficiaries, to raise the eligibility age for receiving Medicare benefits from 65 to 67 years of age, to turn Medicaid into a block grant, and to partially privatize the Social Security system (by allowing contributors to control how their payroll contributions are invested as opposed to using a Federally controlled trust fund). All those efforts have been turned back.

The ability of older persons and their advocacy groups to resist, at least for the moment, those dramatic changes in public benefits for the elderly, reflects a 60-year history of constituent mobilization and interest group politics (Browne and Olson, 1983). The rise of groups such as the American Association for Retired Persons (AARP), National Council on Senior Citizens (NCSC), Gray Panthers and National Council on Aging (NCOA) stems from the 1930s, when senior citizens pushed state legislatures to enact pension protections for impoverished elderly. The Great Depression took a high toll among older persons, especially middle-income elders who lost their retirement savings, homes and livelihood. Their influence pressured President Franklin D. Roosevelt to pass the Social Security Act of 1935, and their ability to participate in presidential politics led to the enactment of Medicare, Medicaid, the Older Americans Act and a host of other benefits (e.g., Supplemental Security Income) and programs (e.g., transportation, housing).

This political clout is a product of a combination of factors: the elderly are more likely to vote than other age groups, they have a sense of interest group solidarity and empowerment, and they are well organized (Peterson and Somit, 1994). Voting patterns among the elderly demonstrate their potent electoral influence. Historically, the elderly have the highest voting rate of any other age group (Binstock, 1997). In 1994, for example, more than 61 percent of the elderly population (age 65 and over) voted, compared with 16 percent of persons between 18 and 20 years of age (U.S. Bureau of the Census, 1994).

Older persons are not necessarily conservative or liberal, however. Their positions on policy issues and their electoral voting patterns reflect their particular cohort. For example, those who were raised during the Depression tend to support federal programs but are socially conservative. As we age, however, and we face the consequences of old age, such as frailty, dependence and impoverishment, group solidarity moves toward protecting benefits and programs (e.g., reducing property taxes, protecting capital gains, preserving Medicare and Social Security). All of these factors make it easier to organize older persons at the local, state and federal levels and to impress upon elected officials that a large portion of their constituents are paying close attention to how politicians address their issues. Thus, the elderly and their organizations wield tremendous influence with municipal government, state legislatures and the Congress. They may not always win, but their views are taken seriously (Torres-Gil, 1992).

Is it possible then to expect that Hispanic elderly might also be a political force? If we assume that social policy could use more allies and that social welfare advocates should build coalitions that enhance their collective influence, then we need to examine who might be the emerging demographic groups from which political influence and voter participation might increase the opportunity to successfully influence political decisions.

In American society today, two of the fastest growing interest groups are Hispanics and the elderly. The Census Bureau predicts that, in 2050, America will be 50 percent more populous than it was in 1995. The largest growth will be in the nation's Hispanic and elderly populations, each of which will represent almost 20 percent of the country's makeup (Newsweek, 1997). Thus, we may ask, might older persons in the Hispanic community be an emerging political force? And if so, can advocates begin now to cultivate those groups and build common agendas with them?

DEMOGRAPHIC TRENDS AND IMPERATIVES

America is aging rapidly. The number of older persons age 65 and older grew from 3 million at the turn of the century to 31 million in 1990 (U.S. Bureau of the Census, 1980 and 1990). In the next three decades, the elderly population will reach 70 million–20 percent of the general U.S. population. The growth of the Hispanic population has also reached a historical high. By 2000, the Hispanic population may increase to 31 million, double its 1990 size. By 2025, there will be 53 million Hispanics–a two-fold increase from 1990–making Hispanics the fastest growing ethnic population and the largest non-white minority group.

Given the growth of the older population in general and Hispanics in particular, what are the projected trends for older persons in the Hispanic community? Currently, of the 1 million elderly Hispanics in the United States, approximately 64 percent are Mexicans, 11 percent are Puerto Ricans, and 5 percent are Cubans (U.S. Bureau of the Census, 1990). While these elderly Hispanics account for only 6 percent of the total Hispanic population and 3.7 percent of the U.S. elderly population–reflecting a relatively young ethnic group–the demographic profile will soon change as Hispanics age and enjoy increased life expectancy. The number of elderly Hispanics will reach 4.7 million by 2020 and 12.5 million by 2050, at which time they will represent 15.5 percent of the U.S. elderly population, compared with Asians at 7 percent, African-Americas at 10.4 percent and non-Hispanic whites at 67 percent (U.S. Bureau of the Census, 1996). Between 1990 and 2030, the number of older Hispanics will increase by 555 percent, compared with 231 percent for native Americans, 169 percent for African Americans and 93 percent for non-Hispanic whites. The growth of the elderly Hispanics will be surpassed only by that of Asian elderly, which will increase by 693 percent.

As these projections demonstrate, the Hispanic elderly will be a dramatically larger portion of the Hispanic population and a substantial proportion of the general elderly population. But herein lies the dilemma: Do they vote? Do they have the potential to be an electoral and political force? The debates over welfare reform, at least publicly, have made it seem that they are a passive, politically invisible and vulnerable population, dependent on sympathetic politicians and advocates to represent their concerns.

ELECTORAL PARTICIPATION

The Hispanic population is becoming an increasingly important part of the political landscape. As Table 1 shows, they accounted for 8.8 percent of the U.S. population in 1992 and represented a diverse set of Latino sub-populations.

In the overall voting population, 3.7 percent were Hispanics, showing that, in fact, they are a relatively small part of the electorate. There are various reasons for this, including the fact that they are a relatively young population with lower levels of education and higher levels of poverty, they do not have a long history of civic involvement in the United States (with important exceptions), and a sizable portion are persons who do not speak English and are undocumented (DeSipio, 1996a).

Nevertheless, the Hispanic vote is becoming increasingly important in certain states. As Table 2 demonstrates, in 1992, Hispanics accounted for 25.5 percent of the vote in New Mexico, 13.6 percent in Texas, 9.6 percent in California and 9.0 percent in Arizona. Given the projected increase in the Hispanic population over the next 20 to 30 years, we can expect that the percentage will increase.

More germane to this discussion are the voting rates of the Hispanic population by age. Figures 1 and 2 illustrate the voting patterns in the 1990 and 1992 elections between Hispanics and non-Hispanic whites.

VOTING RATE

Older Hispanics are more likely to vote than their younger cohorts. For example, in the 1990 election, 44 percent of older Hispanics between ages 65

TABLE 1. National Overview on Hispanic Population and Voting Rate

	United States 1992
Population	251,447,000
Hispanic population	22,096,000
% Hispanics in the total population	8.8
% Mexican Americans in the Hispanic population	63.6
% Puerto Ricans in the Hispanic population	10.6
% Cuban Americans in the Hispanic population	4.7
% Other Hispanics in the Hispanic population	21.2
Voting population	113,866,000
Hispanic voters	4,238,000
% Hispanics in the voting population	3.7
Hispanic adult non-citizens	5,910,000
Electoral votes	538

Source: Adapted from de la Garza, R. O., and DeSipio, L. (1996). *Ethnic Ironies: Latino Politics in the 1992 Elections*. Boulder, CO: Westview Press, p. 1.

and 74 voted, compared with only 10 percent of those between 18 and 20 years of age (Figure 1). In addition, two other age groups–75 years and over and 55 to 64 years of age–had the second and third highest voting rate of 33 and 34 percent, respectively. Combining the three highest voting age groups–persons age 55 and older–2.2 million persons were represented, or 16.5 percent of the Hispanic voting age population in 1990.

In 1992, a similar pattern held among older Hispanics, where 42 percent of those between 65 and 74 years of age voted, compared with only 16 percent of those between 18 and 20 years of age (Figure 2). Persons between 55 and 64 years of age and those who were 75 years and over had the next highest voting rates, at 45 percent and 36 percent, respectively. And together, the three oldest age groups–those age 55 and older–accounted for approximately 2.4 million individuals, or about 16.7 percent of the voting age population among Hispanics.

In analyzing the data, however, the voting rates were lower among His-

TABLE 2. Latino Share of the 1992 Statewide Vote in Selected States

State	Total Vote	Latino Vote	% Latino of statewide vote
Arizona	1,728,000	156,000	9.0
California	11,789,000	1,135,000	9.6
Colorado	1,688,000	136,000	8.1
Florida	5,772,000	411,000	7.1
Illinois	5,650,000	171,000	3.0
New Jersey	3,572,000	173,000	4.8
New Mexico	675,000	172,000	25.5
New York	7,613,000	382,000	5.0
Texas	6,817,000	927,000	13.6

Source: Adapted from Desipio, L. (1996b). *Counting on the Latino Vote: Latinos as a new electorate*. Charlottesville, VA: University of Virginia Press, p. 69. Data from the U.S. Bureau of the Census. (1993). *Voting and Registration in the Election of November 1992*. Current Population Reports, Population Characteristics Series P-20 No. 466. Washington, DC: U.S. Government Printing Office.

panics in general than those of non-Hispanic whites. Despite this difference, voting patterns were consistently the same regardless of race–the older the age group, the higher the voting percentage. One exception was that Hispanics 75 and older showed a lower voting rate than persons age 65 to 74. This is not unusual; it happens with non-Hispanic whites as well. The lower rate reflects the frailties of old age. Even then, this age group is more likely to vote than persons younger than 55 years of age in 1990. In summary, Hispanics age 55 and over are more likely to vote within their ethnic group and thus may be in a position to play a significant role in the electoral power of the Hispanic community.

POLITICS OF AGING IN THE HISPANIC COMMUNITY

These data demonstrate that, of the Hispanic population that participates in electoral politics, it is the older segment that is voting. Therefore, Hispanic older persons are an important part of the electorate within the Latino community. The extent to which this is recognized by Hispanic elected officials is unclear. A literature review does not turn up studies or surveys on this subject. Anecdotally, however, we can surmise that Hispanic city council members, state legislators and congressionally elected officials are well

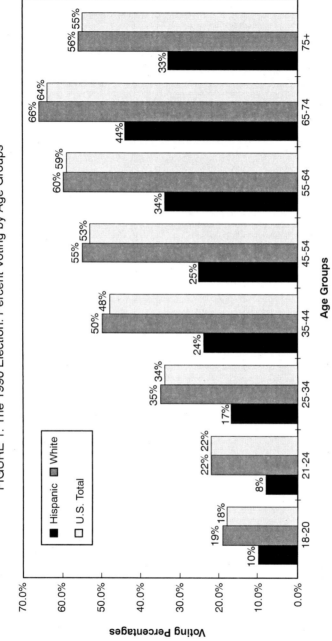

FIGURE 1. The 1990 Election: Percent Voting by Age Groups

Source: U.S. Bureau of the Census, Current Population Reports: Voting and Registration in the Election of November, 1990, Series P-20, #453, pp. 16-17, Table 2. C 3.186/3-2:992.

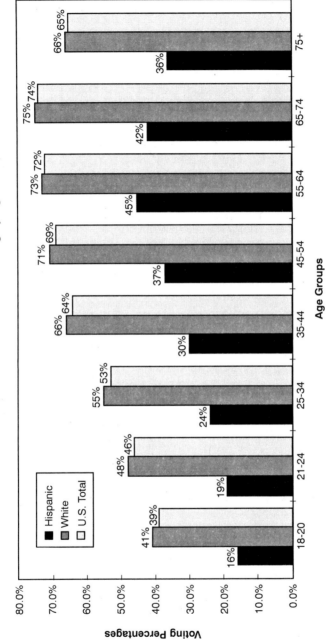

FIGURE 2. The 1992 Election: Percent Voting by Age Groups

Age Groups

Voting Percentages

Source: U.S. Bureau of the Census, Current Population Reports: Voting and Registration in the Election of November, 1992, Series P-20, #466, pp. 4-5, Table 2. C 3.186/3-2:992.

aware that Hispanic senior citizens are a potent segment of their constituencies. One has only to visit senior citizen centers during election time to know that elected officials–Hispanic and non-Hispanic–take this vote seriously.

The larger issue, however, is whether established advocacy groups concerned about social issues and social welfare recognize Hispanic elders as a constituency that engages in political activities. To what extent are Hispanic older voters sought out as potential partners? The answer is probably not much. In part, Hispanic elders are not organized like older persons in general. There are no major Hispanic old-age groups similar to the American Association of Retired Persons (AARP). Hispanic senior citizen groups exist in most communities with large Hispanic populations, but they are usually not actively engaged in organized electoral activities. The two national organizations purporting to represent Hispanic elders–the National Hispanic Council on Aging and the Asociacion Nacional Pro Personas Mayores–are non-profit groups that provide social services and policy advocacy. Established organizations like the AARP do not specifically purport to represent Hispanics, although their large memberships undoubtedly includes some Hispanics.

In addition, the myths and perceptions of Hispanic elders do not easily distinguish between those who are citizens and those who are not. The Welfare Reform Bill affected only legal immigrants, large numbers of whom are Central Americans and Mexicans (as well as Asians, Armenians, and Russian Jews), yet public and media attention talked about Hispanic elderly as if all Hispanic elders were not citizens. In fact, most Hispanic elders are already citizens, whether native-born or naturalized. But even among those who are non-citizens, naturalization rates appear to be increasing. Having an overview of the current state of non-citizens and the naturalization process would allow one to project the potential influences and complexities of political participation among Hispanics and how newly naturalized Hispanics (and Hispanic elderly) might add to the considerable electoral participation of Hispanic elders.

Non-Citizens

Non-citizens, both legal immigrants and undocumented residents, can potentially become constituents. Since the 1980s, Hispanics have made up a large proportion of both legal immigrants and undocumented residents. Given that a large number of the legal immigrants may be eligible for the naturalization process and that there are efforts to naturalize eligible residents, the power of political participation among Hispanics may come sooner than expected. The following data obtained from the Department of Immigration and Naturalization Services (INS) provide evidence that non-citizens, if naturalized, will add to the potential electoral pool.

Legal Permanent Residents

As of April 1996, 10.5 million legal permanent residents resided in the United States (INS), about 4 percent of the U.S. population. In 1996, approximately 32 percent of the legal permanent residents were Hispanics–persons whose country of origin is Spanish-speaking (INS, 1996). The leading Spanish-speaking countries of origin were Mexico (18 percent), Cuba (3 percent), El Salvador (2 percent), Colombia (2 percent) and Peru (1 percent).

Undocumented Residents

In 1996, the INS estimated that there were 5.4 million undocumented residents living in the United States, an equivalent of 2 percent of the U.S. population. The undocumented tend to concentrate in certain regions. For example, California has the highest proportion, about 40 percent of the undocumented residents. Mexico is the leading country of origin with 2.7 million, or 54 percent. Since 1988, approximately 150,000 undocumented Mexicans have arrived in the United States every year.

Naturalization

The INS estimates that approximately 5.8 million people–half of the permanent resident population–are eligible to apply for U.S. citizenship. Although the actual naturalization rate varies by age and country of origin, it has increased in recent years, in large part because of fears among non-citizens about losing public benefits. The number of naturalized persons has increased from 270,000 in 1990 to approximately 1.1 million in 1996. The INS anticipates an additional increase of more than 1 million over the next three years (INS, 1997a). About 30 percent of the persons naturalized were from the Caribbean, Central and South America, and Mexico. Mexico alone composed 6 percent of the naturalized population in 1990. Given this figure, approximately 2 million Hispanics are eligible for naturalization. If we assume that 20 percent of that number are 55 years of age or older, then approximately 400,000 elderly Hispanics will be potential citizens. This does not include the undocumented residents who may add to this potential pool of legal residents and citizens.

Naturalization Process for the Elderly

Before non-citizens can vote, of course, they must be naturalized and registered. The naturalization process can be a daunting process. It requires both specific knowledge–English language proficiency and knowledge of U.S.

civics and history–and the ability to meet various bureaucratic requirements. For example, according to the INS published guidelines, one must be "18 years of age or older; be a legal permanent resident for at least 5 years or 3 years if married to a U.S. citizen, be a person of good moral character, be able to speak, read, write and understand ordinary English words and phrases, and be able to demonstrate knowledge and understanding of the fundamentals of U.S. history and principles of government." For an ordinary older adult who has immigrated late in life, overcoming the anxiety associated with the complicated naturalization process as well as a feeling of detachment away from his or her country of origin, can be daunting. Two requirements, in particular, an English language examination and a civics examination, deter many elderly from applying for citizenship, given their limited English skills and knowledge about the U.S. history and culture.

Recent efforts, however, have streamlined those requirements for older and disabled immigrants. For example, according to the 1997 INS guidelines, people who are 55 years old with a 15-year legal stay in the U.S. are exempt from the language test (INS, 1997b). In California, those elderly immigrants are allowed to take a written test after the completion of a citizenship class and to be interviewed in their native language. Thus, there is a real potential that naturalization rates will continue to increase among immigrants, young and old, adding to the potential pool of older voters in the Hispanic community.

POLITICAL AND RESEARCH AGENDA

Assuming that the pool of Hispanic voters increases, to what extent they will come together on a common agenda and be willing to build coalitions with other groups such as minorities, women, disabled, and social advocates, is an open question. For example, what issues or concerns lead them to participate in the U.S. political system? Are they issues germane to all Americans, to Hispanics, to the elderly, or to themselves as individuals? Added to these dynamics is the unclear effect of acculturation and assimilation on voting patterns and voting behaviors. However we speculate about these scenarios, Hispanic older persons already display a level of political efficacy commensurate with older persons in general by having the highest voting rates. Thus, the challenge for researchers, advocates, policy makers, and elected officials is how to bring this activism into the political and electoral process and around a set of agendas that promote the social welfare of this and other vulnerable groups.

The data show that the politics of aging in the Hispanic community is emerging, albeit with many unanswered questions requiring much more research and analysis. As mentioned earlier, the literature on Hispanic elderly and political participation is quite limited (Bass et al., 1990). More information is needed to gain a comprehensive picture of the dynamics of voter participation. The available data is quite generic and does not allow for a precise understanding of the potential of political participation by Hispanic elders. To do so requires data and information that allow for stratification by:

- Hispanic elders who are native born;
- Hispanic elders who are naturalized;
- Amount of time Hispanic elders are in the U.S.;
- Hispanic elders who are legal immigrants;
- Hispanic elders who are illegal immigrants;
- The Hispanic elders population by country of origin; and
- Hispanic elders by education, income and language fluency.

In the absence of this information, we can only speculate about the potential to organize, register and naturalize Hispanic older persons, which in the aggregate will reveal the true potential to consider Hispanic elders as a potent political force, ready to be courted and involved in social and political objectives.

The fact that we have data on electoral and political activities of older Hispanics causes other issues to surface: To what extent can they, as an organized interest group, be an effective political ally? As mentioned earlier, they do not yet have a history of old-age politics. This may change in time. As they grow older, and as they develop a cohort identification with older persons, they may well develop political agendas that focus on preserving benefits to older persons. In particular, Social Security and Medicare are important programs to Hispanic elders and their families, given the higher rates of poverty in the Hispanic community, especially among older Hispanics. Issues of caregiving and long-term care become important to families caring for older relatives (Angel and Angel, 1997). As long as Medicaid continues its focus on institutional care to the exclusion of home- and community-based care, Hispanic families and elders will find a natural alliance with older persons in general and with persons with disabilities, both of whom are equally concerned about how they take care of others and are taken care of.

In addition, another cohort will soon make its mark on electoral politics and the Hispanic community–the aging of Hispanic baby boomers. Much debate and discussion is occurring about the aging of the post-World War II generation–a group that will more than double the number of older persons from today's 30 million to approximately 70 million by the year 2030 (Light, 1988). Approximately 8.9 percent of this group are members of the Hispanic cohort. How will they impact politics, and to what extent will they see themselves as members of an old-age group engaged in the politics of aging?

Much work and research is required to obtain a clear picture of the demographic, social and political trends facing the Latino community as it ages. That the Hispanic population will be an important part of American society in the next century is indisputable. What remains unclear, however, is the extent to which middle-aged and older Hispanics will have an influence on the issues that matter to them as retirees and senior citizens. This article attempts to shed initial light on the potential voting influence of older Hispanics and to encourage more investigation into the politics of aging in the Hispanic community.

REFERENCES

Angel, R. and Angel, J. (1997). *Who Will Care for Us? Aging and Long Term Care in Multicultural America*. New York, NY: University Press.

Bass, S., Kutza, E., and Torres-Gil, F. (eds.) (1990). *Diversity in Aging. Glenview*, IL: Scott, Foresman and Company.

Binstock, R. (1997). "The 1996 Elections: Older Voters and Implications for Policies on Aging." *The Gerontologist*, vol. 37, no. 1, 15-19.

Browne, W., and Olson, L. (eds.) (1983). *Aging and Public Policy: The Politics of Growing Old in America*. Westport, CT: Greenwood Press.

Desipio, L. (1996a). "Making citizens or good citizens? Naturalization as a predictor of organizational and electoral behavior among Latino immigrants." *Hispanic Journal of Behavioral Science*, vol. 18, no. 2. May, 194-213.

Desipio, L. (1996b). *Counting on the Latino Vote: Latinos as a new electorate.* Charlottesville, VA: University of Virginia Press, p. 69.

Immigration and Naturalization Services (1996). *Immigration to the United States in Fiscal Year 1996.* Available from http://www.ins.usdoj.gov/public/stats/1005.html.

Immigration and Naturalization Services (1997a). *Welfare Reform Questions and Answers.* Available from http://www.ins.usdoj.gov/hqopp/qsandas.html.

Immigration and Naturalization Services (1997b). *Frequently Asked Questions,* Available from http://www.ins.usdoj.gov/faq/93.html.

Light, P. (1988). *Baby Boomers.* New York, NY: W.W. Norton and Company.

Newsweek. (1997). "Living in the 21st century." *Newsweek*, vol. 27, January, 57-59.

Peterson, S. and Somit, A. (1994). *The Political Behavior of Older Americans.* New York, NY: Garland Publishing.

Torres-Gil, F. (1982). *Politics of Aging among Elder Hispanics.* Washington, DC: University Press of America.

Torres-Gil, F. (1992). *The New Aging: Politics and Change in America.* Westport, CT: Auburn House.

U.S. Bureau of the Census. (1980). Census of Population, PC80-B1, Tables 42 and 45, *General Population Characteristics.* Washington DC: U.S. Government Printing Office.

U.S. Bureau of the Census. (1986). *Current Population Reports*, Series P-25, No. 995, *Projections of the Hispanic Population: 1983 to 2080.* Washington DC: U.S. Government Printing Office.

U.S. Bureau of the Census. (1990). Census of Population and Housing, Series CPH-L-74, *Modified and Actual Age, Sex, Race, and Hispanic Origin Data*. Washington DC: U.S. Government Printing Office.

U.S. Bureau of the Census. (1994). November 1994 Congressional election voting and Registration. www.census.gov/population/www/socdemo/voting/vote-tabtcon.html.

U.S. Bureau of the Census. (1996). Current Population Reports, Special Studies, P23-190, *65+ in the United States*. U.S. Government Printing Office, Washington D.C.

Ethnic Differences
in the Expression of Caregiver Burden:
Results of a Qualitative Study

Vanessa Calderón, MS, MA
Sharon L. Tennstedt, PhD

SUMMARY. African American caregivers regularly report less burden than their White counterparts. Less is known about levels of burden among Puerto Rican caregivers. Yet both of these ethnic minority groups tend to provide more hours of care to their elders, mostly due to higher levels of functional disability among ethnic minority elders. A qualitative study was undertaken to detect differences in the way caregivers in three ethnic groups (African American, Puerto Rican and White) describe their experiences with and reactions to caregiving. Caregivers were selected from the larger sample of the Springfield Elder Project, a study of a population-based sample of older adults and their caregivers. Ethnic and gender differences were detected both in how caregivers in the three groups describe the caregiving experience and how they cope with it. White females, and African American and Puerto Rican males expressed feelings of frustration and anger during difficult times in their caregiving situations. Women, particularly African Americans and Puerto Ricans, used somatic complaints as outlets for those feelings. In addition, African American caregivers described their caregiving as an extremely time-consuming activity. Puerto Rican female caregivers described their caregiving situation as one which fos-

---

Vanessa Calderón and Sharon L. Tennstedt are affiliated with New England Research Institutes, 9 Galen Street, Watertown, MA 02172.

This research was supported by the National Institute on Aging Grant No. AG11171.

[Haworth co-indexing entry note]: "Ethnic Differences in the Expression of Caregiver Burden: Results of a Qualitative Study." Calderón, Vanessa, and Sharon L. Tennstedt. Co-published simultaneously in *Journal of Gerontological Social Work* (The Haworth Press, Inc.) Vol. 30, No. 1/2, 1998, pp. 159-178; and: *Latino Elders and the Twenty-First Century: Issues and Challenges for Culturally Competent Research and Practice* (ed: Melvin Delgado) The Haworth Press, Inc., 1998, pp. 159-178. Single or multiple copies of this article are available for a fee from The Haworth Document Delivery Service [1-800-342-9678, 9:00 a.m. - 5:00 p.m. (EST). E-mail address: getinfo@haworthpressinc.com].

159

tered social isolation. Resignation, denial, respect and faith in religion were ways these caregivers dealt with the burden of their caregiving responsibilities. These findings suggest that African American and Puerto Rican caregivers are experiencing burden, but expressing it in different ways than White caregivers and that available measures of caregiver burden do not adequately measure the impact of caregiving on minority caregivers. *[Article copies available for a fee from The Haworth Document Delivery Service: 1-800-342-9678. E-mail address: getinfo@ haworthpressinc.com]*

INTRODUCTION

The investigation of caregiver burden has received much attention in the gerontological literature. Typically, it is assumed that caring for a very disabled elder is stressful for a caregiver, although recently the positive effects of this caregiving have also been acknowledged (Dorfman, Holmes & Berlin, 1996; Haley, Clair & Saulsberry, 1992; Walker, Shin & Bird, 1990; White-Means & Thornton, 1996). Consistently reported from studies to date are differences between White and ethnic minority caregivers in the level of burden associated with the care provided to an older relative. Most studies comparing caregiver burden among different ethnic groups have looked at African Americans and Whites. Overall, in these studies, African American caregivers regularly report less burden than their White counterparts (Aranda & Knight, 1997; Connell & Gibson, 1997; Fredman, Daly & Lazur, 1995; Haley, West, Wadley, Ford, White, Barrett, Harrell & Roth, 1995; Hinrichsen & Ramírez, 1992; Lawton, Rajagopal, Brody & Kleban, 1992; Morycz, Malloy, Bozich & Martz, 1987; Mui, 1992; Stueve, Vine & Struening, 1997). The reasons for this remain unclear since minority elders show higher levels of disability and, therefore, greater need for informal care (Angel & Hogan, 1994; Hinrichsen & Ramírez, 1992; Lacayo, 1980; Wallace, Levy-Storms & Ferguson, 1995). Therefore, we might expect higher levels of burden among minority caregivers due to lower functional status among these elderly.

Less is known about caregiver burden among Latinos. Previous research shows that Latino adult children behave differently toward their parents than do African Americans or Whites (Cox & Monk, 1990; Pacheco & Manaster, 1988). For example, Latinos are more likely than African Americans to report that it is expected of them to help their older parents. Similarly, Latino adult children express that it is important to live close to their parents, in order to provide assistance when needed (Cox & Monk, 1990). However, in terms of burden, there is inconclusive evidence on how these groups may differ. Cox & Monk (1990) reported that both African American and Latino caregivers, mostly Puerto Ricans, were similar in terms of levels of burden.

However, Latino caregivers showed higher levels of depression than African Americans. In a subsequent study of caregivers of elders with Alzheimer's disease, Cox & Monk (1996) found higher levels of strain among Latino caregivers as compared to African Americans. Nevertheless, older Latinos in this study were also more impaired, both in disturbed behavior and in functional disability, which left those caregivers in a more stressful situation. Yet in a study comparing Cuban American and White caregiver daughters of Alzheimer's patients, there were no significant differences in the level of depression (Mintzer, Rubert, & Herman, 1994). However, the sample was very small (N = 28). The only study which compared caregivers across all three ethnic groups–Latinos, Whites and African Americans–looked at informal providers of care to adults with serious mental illness (Stueve et al., 1997). In this study, Latinos and Whites reported similar levels of burden, whereas African American caregivers reported less burden.

Potential explanations have been offered for these differences in the levels of burden among different ethnic groups. First, the family represents the major source of informal caregivers for the elderly. The sense of familial responsibility is assumed to be higher among minorities than among Whites, which could result in a greater sense of obligation to provide care for older family members (Chilman, 1993; Cox & Monk, 1990; García-Preto, 1982; Hurtado, 1995; Mintzer et al., 1994; Sánchez-Ayéndez, 1989). These feelings of obligation may, in turn, affect the expression of burden by the Latino and African American caregivers. In other words, this sense of obligation may translate into the acceptance of the caregiving situation without feeling able to describe it as stressful or burdensome. Second, it has been argued that the often larger extended family of ethnic minority groups, including both relatives and friends, plays an important role in the caregiving situation. This larger support network is thought to ease the responsibilities for the primary caregiver, thereby accounting for the lower levels of burden.

In this paper, we pose a third possibility–that the reported ethnic differences in caregiver burden are a result of measurement. It is possible that ethnic groups differ in the way they respond to measures of burden, even though they might be experiencing similar levels of burden, due to cultural factors that impede expression or admission of burden. Several scales have been developed to measure burden and to study its impact. However, there are various difficulties with these scales. First, a major problem has been the different conceptual definitions of burden and related variables. There is not a clear demarcation on whether caregiving is defined as burden itself, or whether burden is a consequence of caregiving (Montgomery, Stull & Borgatta, 1985). Furthermore, as burden is affected by different factors of the caregiving situation–level of disability of the elder, age and gender of the caregiver, relationship of the caregiver, and financial impact, sharing the same household, among others–there is more than one way a caregiver may be burdened. Secondly, these scales have used different approaches to measure burden, whether they measure objective or subjective burden, or whether they measure both. Finally, the applicability of the different measures to different populations of caregivers and care recipients poses another problem. Most of the measures have been developed to assess the level of burden among caregivers who provide care to elders with Alzheimer's disease, or other types of dementias. In other words, many measures have been developed with a particular care recipient population in mind; however, they have been applied to populations with different conditions.

These methodological problems with the measurement of burden have likely contributed to inconsistent findings (Braithwaite, 1992; Vitalino, Young & Russo, 1991). Furthermore, none of these measures has accounted for cultural differences that are inherent within ethnic minority groups. In other words, these scales are color blind, implying that there are no ethnic differences in the feelings and experiences that caregivers of other ethnic groups face on a daily basis. Instruments and scales that have been developed and standardized on the dominant culture samples have limited value in gathering data on other cultural group samples (Rogler, 1989).

Would the fact that African American and Puerto Rican caregivers show lower levels of burden as compared to their White counterparts be a result of measurement? Are currently available measures of caregiver burden sensitive enough to identify burden in these ethnic groups? Is it possible that these caregivers are experiencing burden, but expressing it in ways that these measures are not able to capture? One thing we are sure of, these caregivers provide more hours of care, on average, than their White counterparts, and the elders for whom they care show higher levels of disability. Therefore, we would expect higher or similar levels of burden among them, but findings to date do not support this assumption.

The goal of this study was to explore how Puerto Rican, African American and White caregivers describe the caregiving experience, how caregivers in each group express feelings of burden, and what coping mechanisms were used to deal with those feelings. In particular, we were interested in whether there were differences in the way each group expressed caregiving burden, and whether these experiences of burden differed from the content of existing measures of caregiving burden. The use of qualitative in-depth interviews allowed caregivers to talk openly about their feelings regarding their caregiving situation and to discuss the sources of potential stress without imposing the constraints of closed-ended questions or rating scales that comprise existing measures of caregiving burden.

METHOD

The sample for this study was drawn from the larger sample of the Springfield Elder Project–a population based study conducted in the city of Springfield, Massachusetts from 1992-1996. The goal of the parent study was to investigate the needs for assistance with daily living activities and the sources and patterns of this help within and between White, African American and Puerto Rican elders age 60 and over. The sample was identified using two sampling frames–the Medicare Enrollment Database and the local annual census list. A total of 977 elders were determined to be frail, or functionally disabled, if they reported difficulty in performing at least one ADL or IADL. Of these disabled elders, 455 reported having an informal caregiver, and 409 caregivers were interviewed.

A stratified random sample of caregivers for this study was selected from the sample of 409 caregivers based on three factors: ethnicity, gender, and coresidence with the care recipient. These factors were selected for the following reasons. First, we wanted to interview caregivers from the three ethnic groups represented in the larger sample by gender and coresidence with the elder. Second, primary informal caregivers are predominantly females (Stone et al., 1987). Nevertheless, we wanted to get the point of view of male caregivers, which are reportedly different from females. And third, caregivers coresiding with the elder often provide more care than those who do not coreside (Tennstedt, Crawford & McKinlay, 1993) and therefore might be more burdened.

Caregivers in this study had no prior acquaintance with each other. They were contacted by telephone, and screened for the above three factors. Individual interviews were scheduled for eligible respondents. All interviews, except for one, were conducted in the caregiver's home–one was conducted in the elder's home. We interviewed a total of 18 caregivers: 4 Whites, 6 African Americans, and 8 Puerto Ricans. Attempts were made to interview the same number of caregivers, at least 8, per ethnic group. Reasons for not achieving this goal among African Americans and Whites include: ineligibility of the elder or the caregiver (e.g., elder deceased, caregiver no longer providing care), inability to establish contact with caregiver (e.g., phone disconnected, moved out of Springfield area), and refusals.

The age of the caregivers in our sample range from 29 to 82 years old, with a mean age of 54.3 years. These caregivers had been providing care to their elders for a period of 4 years on average. The number of hours of care provided by these caregivers is important because it could have affected the burden felt and expressed by them. On average, these caregivers provided 49.9 hours of care in the month prior to the quantitative telephone interview. The physical, emotional and cognitive health status of the care recipients account for this considerable amount of care provided by these caregivers.

More than half of this sub-sample of elders showed some degree of cognitive impairment. When broken down by group, 4 African American elders were cognitively impaired, and 3 Puerto Rican and 3 White elders had this type of disability. Similarly, 67% of the African American elders were severely physically impaired (i.e., having difficulty in performing four or more ADLs or IADLs) as compared to 75% of Whites, and 87.5% of Puerto Ricans. Finally, almost half of these elders, regardless of ethnic background, showed moderate levels of depression as measured by the CES-D (Radloff, 1977).

As mentioned above, coresidence can also have an impact on the levels of burden experienced by caregivers. In this sub-sample of 18 caregivers, 10 coresided with the frail elder. Six of these 10 caregivers were spouses (2 Puerto Ricans, 2 African Americans, and 2 Whites); the remaining four coresiding caregivers were 2 daughters (1 Puerto Rican, 1 African American), one African American niece, and one Puerto Rican son.

Based on the Nam-Power Socioeconomic Index (Nam & Power, 1983), the majority of these caregivers were of low to moderate socioeconomic status. Also, the majority (n = 10) was married. All white caregivers were married, and three of each of the other groups were married as well. The majority of the caregivers in our sample reported to be in good or very good health. However, 5 out of the eight Puerto Rican caregivers reported fair health status as compared to one African American and zero Whites.

Intensive (Lofland & Lofland, 1984) or in-depth interviewing (Kaufman, 1994) was the methodology chosen to elicit rich, detailed information about caregiving from these caregivers. This kind of approach, which is a guided-unstructured conversation, combines different aspects including ethnographic, biographical and therapeutic interviewing (Kaufman, 1994). In this study, the ethnographic interview approach was used. Each interview was conversational and non-directive, permitting the participants to talk openly about their caregiving situation within the structure of an interview guide. However, probing beyond the first level of questions elicited more detailed responses about their caregiving situation. The interview guide included questions about a typical day in their caregiving situation, eliciting examples of a good day, examples of a low point in the provision of care, their feelings during those difficult times, and how they dealt with those feelings. All of the interviews were conducted by the first author. The length of the interviews ranged from 35 to 60 minutes. All caregivers agreed to participate and signed an informed consent form (either in Spanish or English), in which the purpose of the study as well as confidentiality was explained. All but two caregivers consented to audiotaping the interview. All audiotaped interviews were transcribed. For the other two interviews, extensive and thorough notes were taken, and a summary was developed immediately after the interview in order to recall as much detail as possible. All Puerto Rican caregivers were interviewed in Spanish. These interviews with Puerto Rican caregivers were transcribed in Spanish and then translated into English by the first author. No discrepancies or problems with semantic equivalence were identified between the two language versions.

Analysis

Data were analyzed using content analysis to discover themes and meanings expressed by these caregivers. A series of separate analytic files (Lofland & Lofland, 1984) were created to classify the different content categories on caregiving burden expressed by these individuals. Efforts were made to keep each category separate and avoid overlap. The approach used for identifying themes was to look at "those statements that are marked in some way as being of great meaning" to the caregivers (Luborsky, 1994, p. 196). Once all of the emergent themes and meanings were identified and categorized, an outline of these categories was created. This outline, eventually, gave shape to this paper.

FINDINGS

Caregivers talked openly about their caregiving situations. Our findings revealed differences in expression of burden, both by ethnicity and gender within ethnicity groups. Generally, caregiving was associated with negative situations and feelings. In this section, we will present themes and expressions of burden as offered by each ethnic group, and they way they cope with those situations.

White Caregivers

Almost all White caregivers, with the exception of the one male in this group, described their situations negatively. They used the words "struggle," "hard," and "difficult" to describe the care they provide. The following quote is from a White caregiver, an only child who provided assistance to her mother who lived alone. In it, she described different circumstances that made her conceive her situation as difficult.

> When we go shopping, it's also another struggle. She always looks for the change she gets to see if it's correct. And there's nothing wrong with that, but she takes so much time, that you can see other people in line like, you know, thinking: 'Please, move on, finish' . . . The other day I was there [mother's house] writing checks, and I wrote one for Blue

Cross/Blue Shield of Mass. She got really mad at me because I wrote Mass, and not Massachusetts. So we had an argument. I finished everything, and got ready to come back home. Then, she started saying: 'Nobody likes me,' or 'You don't like me,' to try to make me stay longer. But it's hard, because you can't reason with her. Sometimes, it just gets to you.

She also expressed feelings of anger and frustration regarding the assistance provided to her mother. According to her, her mother had memory problems and was somewhat "manipulative." Her frustration turned into anger around different situations that happened frequently.

If she has an appointment, I go there to pick her up, and she's usually not ready. So, I always have to wait for her, you know. I really get angry and upset with her . . . Oh, another thing! If I tell her that I'll pick her up at 2:00 P.M., she starts calling here at 5 or 10 of. So, she drives my husband crazy, too. Then I get there and she's not ready. She's like that.

Another White caregiver providing care to her mother described caregiving as "hard." She described multiple role responsibilities–caregiving along with her other responsibilities as the mother of four school-aged children and a wife–and reported physical consequences.

It's giving me ulcers! [Laugh] Literally! [In a more serious tone] . . . It's tough. I don't have a job outside the house, but if I did, I would have to, definitely, [Pause] have to put her in a nursing home.

In fact, women were more likely than men to express burden through somatic complaints, regardless of their ethnic background. As we will report throughout, this phenomenon was observed among all three groups of female caregivers. Female caregivers in this sample reported a variety of somatic symptoms as a result of their caregiving situations including: weight loss, physical weakness, sleeplessness, exhaustion, nervousness, and ulcers. In the above case, the burden of caring for her mother had translated into the onset of ulcers.

A third White female who was taking care of her husband similarly described caregiving as "hard, difficult and tough," also causing her weakness and exhaustion.

It wasn't easy. I don't have a life, a normal life, let's put it that way. When I have to do some shopping, grocery shopping, I wait until the afternoon when he's taking a nap.

In contrast to these caregivers, a male White caregiver described his situation more positively. He was caring for his wife who suffered from arthritis, so it was difficult for her to do housework, and to walk long distances. He said that the assistance provided was minimal and that providing this assistance made him feel helpful and still active. When further probing was used to elicit potential feelings of burden, he reported that even in tough circumstances surrounding his caregiving, he never got "frustrated or angry." He explicitly expressed satisfaction with the caregiving situation mostly because his assistance was minimal and gave him a sense of purpose.

African American Caregivers

African Americans described their caregiving situation as demanding and time-consuming expressing burden through feelings of frustration, anger and somatic complaints. For example, two African American males expressed explicit feelings of *frustration* to describe difficult moments in their caregiving situations. One of these males explained that he thought that after retirement he would have had some time for traveling, and that because of the care he provided to his brother, who lived alone and had memory problems, he had set aside his plans. Furthermore, his caregiving responsibilities made him give up a part-time job he had. He said:

> I feel disappointed, and sometimes frustrated . . . I used to have a part-time job [after retirement] driving those vans for the elderly with special needs . . . I finally left it. If I wouldn't been taking care of my brother, that's what I'd be doing, a part-time job.

Another African American male providing care to his aunt who lived in the same apartment building said that "it gets frustrating" when he had other things to do, and he had to rush to get everything done.

One African American female did not use the word frustration explicitly, but expressed it in a different way. She said: "There are times that I feel: 'AAHHH!' . . . When there is a lot of calling. When she keeps calling me a lot during the day." When asked to describe more specifically how she feels during those times, she just could not put it into words.

In general, African American caregivers described their situation as demanding and time-consuming, even when they were not coresiding with the care recipient. Another caregiver taking care of his wife described his situation, not only as difficult and time-consuming, but also as one that created confusion in the household due the wife's memory problems.

> When I ask, you know, to do this or do that, it becomes very confusing sometimes . . . It's something you can't really put in words with nobody. You do have to live it day to day. You don't want to say it's bad from the time you get up, 'til the time you go to bed, from Sunday to Sunday. It's

not that bad all the time. At times, it's smooth, but it don't last . . .
Trying to make her understand is the worst, worst part.

Among our sample of caregivers, an African American female living and
taking care of her mother, said that when her mother was ill with her heart
problems, she did not sleep. She further explained how sometimes she was so
tired, weak, and depressed that she had to call in sick, since her job was very
demanding–she is a prosecutor–and could not afford to get to work tired.

Caregiving could also be a positive and rewarding experience for African
Americans. A male providing help for his spouse described his caregiving
situation as good. His wife was very independent and most of the help she
needed was with housework. He said that for him helping her had been
"normal; [he did not] find none of those things [he did], too bad." One
African American female defined her caregiving situation as part of her
family obligations and responsibilities toward her aunt.

If someone is sick, and someone can go and help out, that's what we do.
That's the way the family is.

That level of commitment toward the family seemed to be the tie that
provided the satisfaction she expressed in her situation. She acknowledged
that at times it could be difficult but that having her mother with them gave
her a "time that [she] can breathe." The support network, particularly her
mother, had been the "key to [her] sanity." This same level of familial
commitment and support was also observed among all the Puerto Rican
caregivers.

Puerto Rican Caregivers

Puerto Rican caregivers, particularly males, reported that it was difficult to
meet the demands of the care required. A Puerto Rican male providing
assistance to his father who lived alone reported that even though he is used
to it now, it was hard at the beginning because it not only took some time
away from his personal interests, but also because it coincided with his
divorce process.

It was hard at the beginning. [Pause] It was hard at the beginning
because it took away, like I say, my time for my amusement . . . I'm
more used to it, but before it was difficult . . . My marital problems got
together with the problem of taking care of my father, and all that was
too hard for me.

He also described an incident, in which his father mixed up the doctor's
appointment time, as frustrating.

I felt very, very frustrated, because when you are counting on some plans, and they go wrong, could you imagine?

The expression of *anger* about the caregiving situation was also present in the description of these caregivers' feelings. Males who perceived their caregiving situation as negative were more likely to say that they get angry and upset at the care recipient than were females. The above Puerto Rican male who expressed frustration when his father mixed up the appointments reported:

He still does things that exasperate me, that make me a little bit angry . . . Could you imagine how I felt? I could have eaten him alive . . . I told him to leave me alone.

Another Puerto Rican male helping his mother said that although he tried not to get angry because it added extra stress to his existing heart condition, sometimes he could not avoid getting "mad and angry, not at her, you know, but at the situation."

One Puerto Rican female who described her caregiving situation negatively was taking care of her father who lived with her. She implicitly stated an overwhelming feeling of isolation as part of her caregiving responsibilities. As a widow for eight years, she was also concerned about how this situation may affect potential relationships with males, and her future in general.

I always feel like I have to keep an eye on him. If I want to go out, I decide not to do it. I don't like to leave him alone for long periods of time . . . Most of the time you want to go to a friend's house, being there for a while, and not being worried . . . I'd like to have more freedom . . . There have been some prospects but since he's so close to me, I don't know how he's going to react. Because you know that the kids get married, and then you stay alone. So, that worries me.

This woman who described how her social life was restricted due to the care she provided to her father, implicitly expressed frustration. Clearly, the high demands of caregiving time from the person giving the help elicits feelings of frustration.

The word "hard" was used by another Puerto Rican female taking care of her husband, who has suffered a mild stroke and now shows cognitive problems:

Well, up to the date, thank God, I've been able to handle it. It's true that sometimes I'm exhausted, because I say: 'Gee, this is too much for me. It's hard.' But I go on and say: 'What can I do?'

As shown previously with White and African American female caregivers, Puerto Ricans are no exception when it comes down to express burden through somatic behaviors. Indeed, this pattern was observed more often among Puerto Rican female caregivers than among their African American and White counterparts. When asked how she felt regarding her caregiving situation, particularly during a low point, the Puerto Rican female providing help for her father expressed:

> I found myself just too little to deal with him. I see myself insufficient to take care of him . . . Well, I felt, I felt very, um [Pause], very worried. I lost weight, because when I'm nervous like that, I don't eat. I get depressed and anxious.

Another Puerto Rican female taking care of her husband reported that the excess of work with him and around the house makes her feel "exhausted" and physically "weak." In addition, she reported having frequent headaches due to the caregiving responsibilities. She explained that she experiences those feelings on a regular basis, about "every other day, or about three times a week." However, she confessed that she tried not to give these feelings too much thought, because otherwise she would feel that way all the time. This Puerto Rican woman used psychosomatic complaints as common outlets for her feelings. For her, this was a more appropriate way of expressing feelings. Culturally, Puerto Ricans highly value and esteem the role of the mother as the most important function of Puerto Rican women. This is related to the sense of self-sacrifice for her offspring and her family. The performance of caregiving tasks, which is expected from them without complaining explicitly about it, and without giving it too much thought, further enhances their nurturing motherhood role, making them morally and spiritually superior and strong.

Caregiving, however, not always elicits feelings of frustration, anger and burden. In many instances, providing care to an older friend or relative could be a rewarding, satisfactory experience. In our sample, several Puerto Rican caregivers described their caregiving situations as good and satisfactory. These caregivers seemed to have an extended network of support, in which there were other people involved in the care or assistance to the elder. One Puerto Rican woman taking care of her grandmother explained how the family divided up the different tasks associated with the care of the elder. She gave two reasons for being the primary caregiver–proximity and language. She lived upstairs in a two family house, which enabled her to render direct and constant assistance as needed. She also acted as the health care manager for her grandmother, since her grandmother, as well as other members of the family, did not speak English and could not communicate with the health care providers. The fact that caregiving was shared made her role more manageable. She acknowledged that without the help from the rest of the family, it would be difficult for her to provide the assistance her grandmother needed.

> Everything is fine, we divide everything up. One does one thing, the other does another thing, and so forth . . . I don't have any problems, because we divide things among ourselves. If it would be just me, then yes . . . It would be more difficult!

She elaborated by giving the following example:

> If my car breaks down, there are other cars that can be used to do the things I do. There's my sister's, my other aunt's, her son's, and so forth.

A Puerto Rican male who provides some help to his cousin, and who lives in the same apartment building, also described his situation as good. She required minimum assistance, mostly cooking, medications and housework, which he provided. Receiving help from others was also an important factor for him. Transportation to doctor's appointments and shopping was provided by other family members. Once again, the level of outside support from other members of the family was a key element in the definition of satisfaction in the caregiving situation.

Coping with Burden

The fact that burden was experienced and expressed differently by ethnic minority caregivers was supported by differences in how they cope with caregiving burden. Among the caregivers in this qualitative study, coping strategies seemed to be differentiated by the caregivers' ethnic background. Specifically, Puerto Rican and African American caregivers showed coping techniques different from White caregivers. However, coping strategies were very similar between these two ethnic minority groups.

Resignation with the caregiving situation was the most frequently expressed way of coping among Puerto Rican and African American caregivers. These caregivers reported that they had gotten used to their situations, and dealt with it just "one day at a time," as an African American male caregiver put it. "What can I do?" was the rhetoric question many of these caregivers asked themselves, without having a clear answer. For them, the future seemed uncertain, but they were not trying to explain it. Their attitude was to work with the present situation and hope for the best in the future. Puerto Rican caregivers, particularly, coped by leaving the future of their situation in God's hands. A Puerto Rican caregiver assisting her husband alluded to the will of God oftentimes during the interview.

> Well, like I say, it might be God's will, because what can I do? . . .
> Thank God, I've been able to handle it . . . Sometimes I say: 'Lord, give
> me the strength, because he doesn't have anyone else, but she [daugh-
> ter] and I.'

This same woman used denial or downplaying of the situation, as well as
the expectation of caring for him as a responsibility or obligation that only
belonged to her, as coping techniques. Her husband, after a series of minor
strokes, had serious memory problems and speech difficulties. When asked
about the possibility of getting some outside formal help, she replied:

> I'm not interested in having someone to come here and help me, be-
> cause at least he can help himself, like taking his shower . . . He has no
> problems. He sleeps well, eats well. In other words, on that aspect he's
> physically doing good. If it wouldn't be for his blood pressure, and his
> mind [memory problems].

This woman, along with other Puerto Rican and African American caregivers, felt that they should do whatever was needed or expected from them
no matter what the difficulties were. This sense of responsibility toward more
dependent members of the family provided these caregivers with a way of
coping and dealing with their particular situations. Once again, the culturally
expected self-sacrificing role of motherhood came up as a pattern.

Familial obligation, responsibility and support were observed in both ethnic minority groups included in this study. The support provided by the
family to the primary caregiver represented a source of relief and coping for
those with the primary responsibility of providing care for an older member
of the family. An African American female explained how the family was
there to help out when someone was sick. Actually, in this particular case, the
assistance received from an extended support network of family and friends
made caregiving a much more pleasant and satisfying activity for her. Similarly, Puerto Rican primary caregivers expressed that the help and assistance
provided by other members of the family helped ease the difficulties resulting
from caregiving. All but one Puerto Rican caregiver reported having other
family members available to help with the different tasks. However, this
sense of responsibility for family members conflicted with the dominant
culture values. On the one hand, the expectation was to assume the responsibility of care. On the other hand, they lived in a culture which highly values
individualism, and thus, may not understand their point of view and the need
to be the primary source of assistance to their elders.

Finally, "respeto" (respect) was another way Puerto Ricans coped with
their caregiving demands, in particular when the caregiving relationship is
adult children-older parent. "Respeto" is an extremely important value

among Puerto Rican familial, personal and social relationships. It acknowledges the other person's social worthiness and authority. Thus, it preserves the network of close, personal relationships (García-Preto, 1982). Puerto Rican caregivers who were providing assistance to their older parents explained that no matter how difficult the situation may have been, they always treated the elderly with the respect they deserved. This mechanism allowed these individuals to deal with the situation, and accept it as part of the relationship itself. For instance, the Puerto Rican male caregiver who got upset at his father after he mixed up doctor's appointments reported that even though he got very angry at him, he still treated his father with respect.

There are moments in which he exasperates me, sometimes I get furious, but I have to respect him because he's my father.

White caregivers, on the other hand, appeared to take a more hands-on approach to deal with feelings of burden. One White female expressed that she enjoyed working in her garden. She said that the time she spent there helped her release all the negative feelings associated with the care she provided to her mother. In other words, working in the garden was her "therapy." Another White female reported that she belonged to a church group, and that in that way she gets distracted from the caregiving responsibilities. Another coping technique observed among White caregivers, but not minority caregivers, was the reliance on formal services to ease the troubles faced in their day-to-day caregiving activities.

DISCUSSION

In research on informal care, the concept of burden has been widely discussed, defined and measured. However, the range of definitions and measures used in this research has led to inconsistent and inconclusive findings regarding the level of burden reported by caregivers, particularly ethnic minority caregivers. Caregiving burden research done with ethnic minority caregivers has focused, for the most part, on the differences between White and African American caregivers. This body of research shows there is a race difference in reporting burden. African Americans show lower levels of burden even when they provide more hours of care to their elders than Whites. Less is known about Puerto Rican caregivers. We suspected that traditional burden scales do not capture burden among minority caregivers because of cultural differences in dealing with and describing the provision of care to an older member of the family. The purpose of this paper was to explore how Puerto Rican, African American, and White caregivers describe their caregiving situation and the feelings associated with burden, and what coping mechanisms were used to deal with those feelings.

All caregivers, regardless of ethnic background, who provided assistance to high functioning elders, or who had an extensive network of support (i.e., other caregivers, or family members) described their caregiving situation as satisfactory. Those whose caregiving situations differed from the one described above (i.e., higher levels of disability among the elderly, weaker social support network) were more likely to categorize the situation as difficult. However, all White caregivers in this sample had smaller support networks, and the elders they cared for were not as impaired as the minority elders. Yet, they explicitly categorized their situations as difficult and openly expressed strong feelings of burden. Minority caregivers, on the other hand, were more likely to provide care to more disabled elders, but their support network was larger. These caregivers expressed burden more indirectly through frustration, anger, isolation and somatic complaints.

White female caregivers were more likely to express feelings of anger with their situations than were African Americans and Puerto Ricans females. However, males in both ethnic minority groups expressed similar feelings of anger as White female caregivers did. Puerto Rican females, on the other hand, described their situation as one which fostered social isolation, whereas African American caregivers, regardless of gender, described their situation as one demanding lots of their time. Some of these caregivers gave up part-time employment in order to meet the demands of the care provided to the elder.

Frustration was reported frequently by the minority caregivers, especially among males, who expressed feelings of disappointment more directly than females. Males were also more likely to openly express feelings of anger when the "tough gets rough." Women, on the contrary, appeared to express frustration and anger indirectly and through somatic complaints. These complaints served as an outlet for the negative feelings associated with their caregiving responsibilities. This finding is supported by existing literature, especially on Puerto Rican women. Traditionally, Puerto Rican women are assigned a less assertive role in the dominant culture, as well as in their own culture. They are expected to be submissive, and less vocal about their feelings and opinions. In fact, assertiveness is a behavior that is discouraged among Puerto Rican women, both in the island and in the mainland, as part of the culture (Comas-Díaz, 1988). This goes against the dominant culture society in the mainland, which values and encourages assertiveness. These traditional roles have been associated with psychological dysfunction, including depression and other physical ailments (Comas-Díaz, 1988; García-Preto, 1982). In fact, depression–one somatic symptom reported by some Puerto Rican women in this sample–is negatively associated with assertiveness among Puerto Rican women in the United States (Soto & Shaver, 1982). As opposed to men's way of ventilating feelings of anger (i.e., explicitly), these women could be expressing their anger and stress towards the caregiving situation through these somatic complaints.

Females in a male dominated society are expected to repress feelings of anger and oppression. As noted before, ethnic minority women face that social pressure to a greater extent due to cultural values and expectations.

Coping strategies differed, based on the ethnicity of the caregiver. Puerto Ricans and African Americans showed coping techniques that were different from those utilized by White caregivers. For example, resignation, denial and respect were ways in which ethnic minority caregivers dealt with the burden of their caregiving responsibilities. Puerto Ricans, in particular, trusted their Catholic faith by hoping that God would take care of the situation, and therefore, would grant them the strength to continue and to bear the burden.

Previous research shows that African American caregivers show less burden than Whites, with no information on Puerto Rican caregivers. The findings from this qualitative study show that burden is a common problem among caregivers across different ethnic groups. While burden was expressed in different ways among the caregivers interviewed for this study, it was certainly expressed in one way or the other.

In summary, based on our qualitative in-depth interviews with White, African American and Puerto Rican caregivers, we found that across all three groups burden was experienced. But, the ways in which they described their caregiving situations, and the very words they used, differed across ethnic groups. In other words, in our data we found evidence to believe that measures traditionally used in previous research do not adequately capture indications of caregiver burden. Thus, previous levels of caregiver burden in ethnic minority groups, in this case African Americans and Puerto Ricans, might have been underreported.

Our qualitative findings reveal that African American and Puerto Rican caregivers are in fact experiencing burden, but expressing it in ways different than commonly used measures developed with samples of White caregivers. According to our findings, any scale developed to measure burden in African Americans and Puerto Ricans should include questions to capture frustration, anger, isolation, and somatic symptoms experienced by these caregivers. This has some major implications for future research on caregiving burden among ethnic minority populations, including Asians. Before any major quantitative findings on caregiving burden can be considered as significant, standardized measures need to account for ethnic differences.

These findings also have implications for policy and practice as many programs and support group models have been developed to help caregivers to cope with the difficulties of caregiving. However, it is difficult, or virtually impossible, to create programs to address the problem of burden among African Americans and Puerto Ricans when current research shows that these groups experience lower levels of burden than their White counterparts. Existing support programs for ethnic minority caregivers may not be completely effective if cultural differences in coping are not taken into consideration in the design, planning and development of such programs. These findings can assist practitioners to better understand the cultural idiosyncrasies that are important in developing a culturally sensitive action plan. Finally, by recognizing and accurately identifying burden among African American and Puerto Rican caregivers, culturally sensitive programs can be developed to target this segment of the caregiver population who are the most important source of long-term care for minority elderly.

REFERENCES

Angel, J.L. & Hogan, D.P. (1994). The demography of minority aging populations. *Minority elders: Five goals toward building a public policy base.* Washington, DC: Gerontological Society of America.

Aranda, M.P. & Knight, B.G. (1997). The influence of ethnicity and culture on the caregiver stress and coping process: A sociocultural review and analysis. *The Gerontologist, 37,* 342-355.

Barber, C.E. (1988). Correlates of subjective burden among adult sons and daughters caring for aged parents. *Journal of Aging Studies, 2,* 133-144.

Barusch, A.S. & Spaid, W.M. (1989). Gender differences in caregiving: Why do wives report greater burden? *The Gerontologist, 29,* 667-676.

Braithwaite, V. (1992). Caregiver burden–making the concept scientifically useful and policy relevant. *Research on Aging, 14,* 3-27.

Cantor, M. (1983). Strain among caregivers: A study of experience in the United States. *The Gerontologist, 23,* 597-604.

Chilman, C.S. (1993). Hispanic families in the United States: Research perspectives. In H.P. McAdoo (Ed.), *Family Ethnicity: Strength in Diversity* (pp. 141-163). California: Sage Publications, Inc.

Comas-Díaz, L. (1988). Mainland Puerto Rican women: A sociocultural approach. *Journal of Community Psychology, 16,* 21-31.

Connell, C.M. & Gibson, G.D. (1997). Racial, ethnic, and cultural differences in dementia caregiving: Review and analysis. *The Gerontologist, 37,* 355-364.

Cox, C. (1995). Comparing the experiences of Black and White caregivers of dementia patients. *Social Work, 40,* 343-349.

Cox, C. & Monk, A. (1990). Minority caregivers of dementia victims: A comparison of Black and Hispanic families. *The Journal of Applied Gerontology, 9,* 340-354.

Cox, C. & Monk, A. (1996). Strain among caregivers: Comparing the experiences of African American and Hispanic caregivers of Alzheimer' relatives. *International Journal of Aging and Human Development, 43,* 93-105.

Dorfman, L.T., Holmes, C.A. & Berlin, K.L. (1996). Wife caregivers of frail elderly veterans: Correlates of caregiver satisfaction and caregiver strain. *Family Relations, 45,* 46.

Fredman, L., Daly, M.P. & Lazur, A.M. (1995). Burden among White and Black caregivers to elderly adults. *Journal of Gerontology: Social Sciences, 50B,* S110-S118.

García-Preto, N. (1982). Puerto Rican families. In M. McGoldrick, J.K. Pearce & J. Giordano (Eds.), *Ethnicity and Family Therapy* (pp. 164-186). New York: Guilford.

Haley, W.E., Clair, J.M. & Saulsberry, K. (1992). Family caregiver satisfaction with medical care of their demented relatives. *The Gerontologist, 32,* 219.

Haley, W.E., Roth, D.L., Coleton, M.I., Ford, G.R., West, C.A.C., Collins, R.P. & Isobe, T.L. (1996). Appraisal, coping, and social support as mediators of well-being in Black and White family caregivers of patients with Alzheimer's disease. *Journal of Consulting and Clinical Psychology, 64,* 121-129.

Haley, W.E., West, C.A.C., Wadley, V.G., Ford, G.R., White, F.A., Barrett, J.J., Harrell, L.E. & Roth, D.L. (1995). Psychological, social, and health impact of caregiving: A comparison of Black and White dementia family caregivers and noncaregivers. *Psychology and Aging, 10,* 540-552.

Hinrichsen, G.A. & Ramirez, M. (1992). Black and white dementia caregivers: A comparison of their adaptation, adjustment, and service utilization. *The Gerontologist, 32,* 375-381.

Hurtado, A. 1995. Variations, Combinations, and Evolutions: Latino Families in mainland United States. In R. Zambrana (Ed.), *Understanding Latino Families: Scholarship, Policy and Practice* (pp. 40-61). Thousand Oaks, CA: Sage Publications.

Jette, A.M., Crawford, S.L. & Tennstedt, S.L. (1996). Toward understanding ethnic differences in later-life disability. *Research on Aging, 18,* 292-309.

Kaufman, S.R. (1994). In-depth interviewing. In J.F. Gubrium & A. Sankar (Eds.), *Qualitative Methods in Aging Research* (pp. 123-136). Thousand Oaks, CA: Sage Publications.

Lacayo, C.G. (1980). *A national study to assess the service needs of the Hispanic elderly.* Los Angeles, CA: Asociación Nacional Pro Personas Mayores.

Lawton, M.P., Rajagopal, D., Brody, E. & Kleban, M.H. (1992). The dynamics of caregiving for a demented elder among black and white families. *The Journals of Gerontology, 47,* S156-164.

Lofland, J. & Lofland, L.H. (1984). *Analyzing Social Settings: A Guide to Qualitative Observation and Analysis.* Belmont, CA: Wadsworth, Inc.

Luborsky, M.R. (1994). The identification and analysis of themes and patterns. In J.F. Gubrium & A. Sankar (Eds.), *Qualitative Methods in Aging Research* (pp. 189-210). Thousand Oaks, CA: Sage Publications.

Mintzer, J.E., Rubert, M.P. & Herman, K.C. (1994). Caregiving for Hispanic Alzheimer's disease patients: Understanding the problem. *The American Journal of Geriatric Psychiatry, 2,* 32-28.

Montgomery, R.J.V., Stull, D.E. & Borgatta, E.F. (1985). Measurement and analysis of burden. *Research on Aging, 7,* 137-152.

Morycz, R.K., Malloy, J., Bozich, M. & Martz, P. (1987). Racial differences in family burden: Clinical implications for social work. *Gerontological Social Work, 10,* 133-154.

Mui, A.C. (1992). Caregiver strain among black and white daughter caregivers: A role theory perspective. *The Gerontologist, 32,* 203-212.

Nam, C. & Power, M. (1983). *The Socioeconomic Approach to Status Measurement.* Houston, TX: Cap and Gown Press.

Radloff, L.S. (1977). A self-report depression scale for research in the general population. *Applied Psychological Measurement, 1,* 385-401.

Rogler, L.H. (1989). The meaning of culturally relevant research in mental health. *American Journal of Psychiatry, 146,* 296-303.

Sánchez-Ayéndez, M. 1989. Puerto Rican Elderly Women: The Cultural Dimension of Social Support Networks. *Women and Health, 14:*239-252.

Soto, E. & Shaver, P. (1982). Sex-role traditionalism, assertiveness, and symptoms of Puerto Rican living in the United States. *Hispanic Journal of Behavioral Sciences, 4,* 1-19.

Stone, R., Cafferata, G.L. & Sangl, J. (1987). Caregivers of the frail elderly: a national profile. *The Gerontologist, 27,* 616-626.

Tennstedt, S.L., Crawford, S.L. & McKinlay, J.B. (1993). Determining the pattern of community care: Is coresidence more important than caregiver relationship? *Journal of Gerontology: Social Sciences, 48,* S74-83.

Vitaliano, P.P., Young, H.M. & Russo, J. (1991). Burden: A review of measures used among caregivers of individuals with dementia. *The Gerontologist, 31,* 67-75.

Walker, A.J., Shin, H. & Bird, D.N. (1990). Perceptions of relationship change and caregiver satisfaction. *Family Relations, 39,* 147.

Wallace, S.P., Levy-Storms, L. & Ferguson, L.R. (1995). Access to paid in-home assistance among disabled elderly people: Do Latinos differ from Non-Latino Whites? *American Journal of Public Health, 85,* 970-975.

White-Means, S.I. & Thornton, M.C. (1996). Well-being among caregivers of indigent Black elderly. *Journal of Comparative Family Studies, 27,* 109-128.

Patterns of Long-Term Care:
A Comparison of Puerto Rican,
African-American,
and Non-Latino White Elders

Sharon L. Tennstedt, PhD
Bei-Hung Chang, ScD
Melvin Delgado, PhD

SUMMARY. Data from an observational study of a population-based sample of Puerto Rican, African-American, and non-Latino White persons age 60+ were used to investigate ethnic differences in the patterns and sources of care provided to functionally disabled elders. In general, ethnicity was not associated with either the types of care or source of care (informal vs. formal) received when controlling for other factors. Extent of disability was the most consistent correlate of likelihood of receiving certain types of help as well as the amount of help from both informal and formal services. In addition, the pattern of care was related to the relationship and coresidence status of the caregiver. These data challenge assumptions about more extensive and more involved caregiving networks of minority elders. *[Article copies available for a fee from The Haworth Document Delivery Service: 1-800-342-9678. E-mail address: getinfo@haworthpressinc.com]*

Sharon L. Tennstedt and Bei-Hung Chang are affiliated with New England Research Institutes, 9 Galen Street, Watertown, MA 02172. Melvin Delgado is affiliated with Boston University School of Social Work, 264 Bay State Road, Boston, MA 02215.

The authors wish to acknowledge the helpful comments of Sybil Crawford, Margie Lachman, and Alan Jette.

This research was supported by the National Institute on Aging Grant No. AG11171.

[Haworth co-indexing entry note]: "Patterns of Long-Term Care: A Comparison of Puerto Rican, African-American, and Non-Latino White Elders." Tennstedt, Sharon L., Bei-Hung Chang, and Melvin Delgado. Co-published simultaneously in *Journal of Gerontological Social Work* (The Haworth Press, Inc.) Vol. 30, No. 1/2, 1998, pp. 179-199; and: *Latino Elders and the Twenty-First Century: Issues and Challenges for Culturally Competent Research and Practice* (ed: Melvin Delgado) The Haworth Press, Inc., 1998, pp. 179-199. Single or multiple copies of this article are available for a fee from The Haworth Document Delivery Service [1-800-342-9678, 9:00 a.m. - 5:00 p.m. (EST). E-mail address: getinfo@ haworthpressinc.com].

179

A study of ethnic differences in the patterns and sources of care provided to functionally disabled elders is important for several reasons–first, the widely recognized increase in the numbers of old, and especially very old, persons in this country (U.S. Bureau of the Census, 1992) and second, the demographic shift from an Anglo-European society to a multiracial, multicultural society (Zinn, 1995). Not only will there be more old, and likely functionally dependent, persons in this country, but also the proportion will be more racially and ethnically diverse (Day, 1992). Public policy concern with the increasing numbers of older persons of color stems from clear evidence of social and health status differences in these groups. Compared to older white, non-Latino persons, African-Americans and Latinos are of lower socioeconomic status, including greater rates of persons at or below poverty status and with less educational attainment (Taeuber, 1993; Litman, 1991) and in poorer health with higher rates of functional disability (Wallace et al., 1994; Hing and Bloom, 1990; U.S. Bureau of the Census, 1990; Van Nostrand et al., 1993). These differences suggest that the disadvantaged status of most older persons of color is likely to result in greater need for long-term care. We know that, for older White, non-Latino populations, demand/use of services is related to disability and to provision of informal care (cf. Tennstedt et al., 1993).

The majority of research on disabled elders and their receipt of care has been conducted with Anglo populations. More recently attention has been directed to African-Americans (Keith, 1987; Chatters et al., 1985, 1986; Taylor and Chatters, 1991; Mui, 1992; Lawton et al., 1992; Hinrichsen and Ramirez, 1992; Miller et al., 1994, 1995) and Latinos (Cox and Monk, 1990; Wallace et al., 1994, 1995; Miller et al., 1995; Burnette and Mui, 1995). However, the data comparing African-Americans, Latinos and non-Latino Whites are limited, especially regarding the specific types and amounts of help received informally and formally. Available data regarding African-Americans and Latinos are usually in comparison to White persons but not to other ethnic minority groups. An exception is the recent work of Miller and colleagues (Miller et al., 1994, 1995) which has investigated ethnic group differences in source and type of care using national data sets.

Families have been recognized as the primary source of long-term care for functionally disabled elders (Doty, 1986; Stone et al., 1987; Tennstedt, and McKinlay, 1989). Ethnic differences in family structure that might influence provision of this care have been well documented. African-Americans and Puerto Ricans generally have larger families, consisting of a wider range of kin as well as non-blood relatives, than do non-Latino Whites (Hays and Mindel, 1973; Mitchell and Register, 1984; Montgomery and Hirshorn, 1990; Greene and Monahan, 1984; Delgado and Humm-Delgado, 1982). However, this similarity between the two minority groups does not extend to their living arrangements. Older Puerto Ricans are more similar to older Whites in that they are likely to live alone (Cantor, 1975; Soldo, 1985; Lacayo, 1980; Sanchez-Ayendez, 1988) whereas African-American elders are more likely to live in, and head, multigenerational households that include a wider range of kin (Cantor, 1975; Hays and Mindel, 1973; Soldo, 1985; Jackson, 1985; Ford et al., 1990; Mutchler, 1990). Yet all three groups are likely to live in close proximity to children and to see them frequently (Shanas, 1979; Horowitz, 1985; Taylor, 1985; Sanchez-Ayendez, 1988; Tennstedt and McKinlay, 1989).

The modified extended families of African-Americans and Puerto Ricans are thought to increase the informal care resources of older persons in these two groups (Chatters, Taylor, and Jackson, 1985, 1986). Contacts with and participation in church activities, social clubs, and ethnic merchants have also been reported as additional sources of support for both groups (Delgado and Humm-Delgado, 1982; Hatch, 1991). Increased reciprocity between older and younger family members has been reported for both African-Americans and Latinos compared to Whites (Cantor 1979, Jackson, 1980; Sotomayer, 1973; Sanchez-Mayers, 1985; Maldonado, 1985; Hatch, 1991), but less is known about the specific types and amounts of help provided to older persons. Further, the data are inconsistent, reporting both ethnic differences (Hays and Mindel, 1973; Cantor 1979; Mitchell and Register, 1984) and similarities (Mindel et al., 1986). Cantor's (1979) study was the only one to compare African-Americans, Whites, and Latinos and reported that Latinos received the most help, but that African-Americans and Whites received similar amounts of help.

Even less is known about utilization of long term care services, especially community-based services, by minority elders (Kart, 1991). It has consistently been found that older African-Americans and Latinos are less likely than Whites to be institutionalized (Eribes and Bradley-Rawls, 1978; Havlik et al., 1987; Hing, 1987; Ford et al., 1990) even when controlling for disability and income (Burr, 1990). It is also generally thought that older African-Americans and Latinos are lower utilizers of community services (Trevino et al., 1983, 1984; Neighbors and Jackson, 1984; Greene and Monahan, 1984; Starrett et al., 1989; Kart, 1991; Kemper, 1992) although findings are inconsistent. For example, in a comparison of data from the Commonwealth Fund Commission's National Study of Older Latinos with data from the 1988 Longitudinal Study on Aging, Wallace et al. (1995) report similar use of formal services by Latinos and non-Latino Whites. However, the measure of service use in this analysis was limited to the dichotomous use/no use. Intensity of use was not compared which might have masked some group differences. Others have reported within-group differences in service use. For example, some data suggest that African-Americans living in inner cities rely on formal services (Johnson and Barer, 1990) or are more likely to use certain types of services (Mindel et al., 1986) than those in non-urban areas. In the National Study of Older Latinos, Puerto Ricans were more likely than Mexican Americans or Cuban Americans to use community services (Wallace, 1994; Burnette and Mui, 1995).

It is typically assumed that lack of cultural assimilation is a major barrier to use for Hispanics (Wallace and Facio, 1987; Morrison, 1983; Sokolovsky, 1990), but this assumption has little empirical support (Chesney et al., 1982; Lopez-Aqueres et al., 1984; Deyo et al., 1985; Markides et al., 1985, Solis et al., 1990). Sociodemographic and structural factors such as lower educational level, lower income and age, accessibility and outreach, as they relate to barriers to access, also predict lower utilization (Bastida, 1983; Solis et al., 1990; Estrada et al., 1990) and Cantor (1979) has suggested that receipt of informal care appears to be a critical predictor of non-use. The importance of informal care in predicting low utilization of formal services has been reported consistently in studies of older Whites, including our own work (Horowitz, 1985; Soldo et al., 1989; Tennstedt et al., 1990).

In sum, methodological limitations in sampling and measurement and lack of comparability of these factors across studies to date have resulted in inconsistent and incomplete data regarding differences in patterns of informal and formal care between non-Latino Whites, African-Americans, and various Latino groups. Detailed data regarding both types and amounts of care and the factors associated with different patterns of care are required to detect ethnic differences and to identify formal service implications of ethnic contrasts among older Americans.

The growing number of elders of color in the United States makes these communities of great importance for the field of social work. Elders of color also present significant challenges for social workers in the development of culturally competent gerontological services. Latino elders such as Puerto Ricans, in turn, provide the additional challenges associated with service provision in Spanish. Gerontological research should emphasize the importance of looking at Puerto Rican elders, for example, within a context of their African-American, and non-Latino White counterparts.

This study was designed to investigate differences between Latino, African-American, and non-Latino White elders regarding needs for long term care assistance and sources and types of care received to address these needs. Because of the cultural diversity among Latinos (Solis et al., 1990), the study focuses specifically on Puerto Ricans, the second largest group of Latinos in the U.S. (U.S. Bureau of the Census, 1991), and the predominant Latino group in the Northeast (U.S. Bureau of the Census, 1989), in order to avoid obscuring between group differences that could result from variability in Latino culture. This paper reports on between-group differences in the sources (informal vs. formal) and patterns of care provided to Puerto Rican,

African-American, and White elders as well as the predictors of various patterns of care. In addition, implications for social work practice with Puerto Rican elders will be presented, keeping in focus the nature of this collection.

METHODS

Sample

The Springfield Elder Project is a comparative observational study to investigate the needs for assistance with daily living activities and the sources (both informal and formal) and patterns of this help within and between Puerto Rican, African-American, and White elders age 60+. The study was located in Springfield, MA for several reasons: (1) the older population is socioeconomically diverse; (2) the city has sufficiently sized populations of older African-Americans and Latinos; and (3) because the city is a major point of population dispersal for Puerto Ricans, they comprise almost all of the Latino population in the city. This permitted study focus on one Latino subgroup in order to avoid obscuring any between group differences that could result from variability in Hispanic culture.

The population-based sample was identified using two sampling frames–the Medicare Enrollment Data Base (EDB) and the local annual census list. This was necessary because of data limitations in each frame. The local census list was used to identify Puerto Ricans primarily because of lack of identified Hispanic origin in the Medicare EDB and also because of concern with potential undercoverage of Puerto Ricans in the Medicare EDB. Because race and/or ethnicity are not indicated in this census list, Hispanic surnames (as well as non-obvious names of persons known to be Hispanic) were identified manually by the staff of a local Latino service and advocacy agency. Then these names were crossmatched with those in the Medicare EDB to identify any additional Hispanic surnames not included in the census list. The Medicare EDB was used to randomly select the samples of African-American and White persons age 65+. These files list race as "white, black, other." Names were sorted by race, with race being confirmed at time of first contact. Then, to obtain a sample of African-American and White persons age 60-64, the local census list was used because Medicare coverage in this age group is limited to the disabled. Because race was not identified in the census list, screening for race by self-report of the potential African-American and non–Hispanic White respondents in this age group was necessary at time of first contact.

Identification of all Puerto Ricans in Springfield was attempted because of the limited number of persons in this group. The size of this group was used to determine the sizes of the random samples of African-Americans and non-Latino Whites. To be able to do this, the separate samples of African-Americans and non-Latino Whites were randomly ordered and contacted in order until the desired number of respondents was obtained. Respondents in all three groups were contacted simultaneously at similar rates. However, by the time all Puerto Ricans had been identified and contacted, large numbers of African-Americans and non-Latino Whites had been enrolled in the study. Therefore, the sample sizes for each group are not equal as was intended.

A primary concern in constructing a sampling scheme is that samples of key subgroups must be large enough to permit reliable estimation of rates, means, etc., as well as meaningful statistical comparisons among them. This requirement can be troublesome, particularly if some of the subgroups of interest constitute relatively small proportions of the target population, as they do in this study. For example, comparisons of prevalence rates of disability between age groups (60-74 vs. 75+) involve small numbers in the older age group, particularly in the African-American sample. This is related to lower life expectancy in African-Americans (Manton et al., 1979). To obtain an adequate sample from the older age group, as well as to insure comparability in the age distribution for African-American, White, and Puerto Rican elders, the samples of African-American and White elders were stratified on age using two strata (60-74 and 75+). The percentage of randomly sampled African-American and White elders from each of these strata matched the corresponding percentages found in the group of Puerto Rican elders.

Data Collection

A two-stage field design was used. In the *first stage*, data were collected from the older persons. The majority (88%) of interviews were completed by telephone with in-home interviews conducted for the 12% of respondents without a listed telephone number. Respondents were first screened for functional disability. A respondent was considered disabled when s/he reported "substantial difficulty" with at least one of 13 personal activities of daily living (or ADLs, e.g., bathing, dressing, toileting), instrumental activities of daily living (or IADLs, e.g., meal preparation, housecleaning, transportation) or mobility (e.g., walking inside or outside the home). If not disabled, a brief (i.e., 15 minute) interview was conducted, collecting sociodemographic data and information regarding their natural support system to investigate potential sources of informal care. Elders identified as functionally disabled (n = 977; 49.5% of respondents) received a more extensive interview (30 minutes), collecting data regarding their informal caregiving network, the help provided by these caregivers, and their use of formal long term care services.

If receiving informal care, the name, address, and telephone number of the person providing the *most* help (i.e., the primary caregiver) was gathered. Of the 483 disabled elders with caregivers (49.4%), the names of these caregivers were provided by 455 respondents. In the *second stage*, telephone interviews (50 minutes) were conducted with 409 primary informal caregivers (response rate 90.9%). Detailed data regarding the types and amount of help provided were collected from the caregiver. Sociodemographic data about the primary caregiver and other (i.e., secondary) caregivers, cultural factors, the motivation for providing care, and the impact of this care on their lives were also collected.

Dispositions and response rates are displayed in Table 1.

Measures

Variables considered in the analyses included elder characteristics: age, gender, martial status, level of functional disability (number of ADL, IADL, and mobility tasks with which the elder reported substantial difficulty), and social class. Social class was measured by the Nam-Power Socioeconomic Index (Nam and Power, 1983) which ranks primary occupation on a scale of 1-100, based on the level of education and average income associated with that occupation as derived from census data. The following caregiver characteristics were considered: coresidence with elder or not, gender, marital sta-

TABLE 1. Sample Dispositions by Ethnic Group

Dispositions	African-Americans		Puerto Ricans		Whites		Total Sample	
	n	%	n	%	n	%	n	%
Sample Elders								
Screened	962		1129		1471		3562	
Eligible Respondents	682	85.1	591	76.6	702	78.6	1975	80.1
Disabled[a]	324		368		285		977	
Non-Disabled	358		223		417		998	
No Contact	34	4.2	165	21.4	28	3.1	227	9.2
Refusals	86	10.7	16	2.0	163	18.3	265	10.7
Ineligible[b]	160	–	357	–	578	–	1095	–
Sample Caregivers								
Identified	148		208		99		455	
Respondents	131	89.1	194	93.7	84	87.5	409	90.9
Refusals	15	10.2	9	4.4	11	11.5	35	7.8
No Contact	1	0.7	4	1.9	1	1.0	6	1.3
Ineligible[b]	1	–	1	–	3	–	5	–

[a]At least one functional disability
[b]Ineligibles excluded from response rate calculation

tus, employment status, and duration of caregiving. Ethnicity of the care recipient was measured as self-reported Puerto Rican, African-American (defined as non-Latino Black), or White (non-Latino). Because of our interest in the influence of an individual's value and belief system, or culture, on receipt of care, we focused on ethnicity rather than race for purposes of defining the groups of comparison. In addition, the following characteristics of the caregiving situation were considered: number of actively involved caregivers and number of potential caregivers. Finally, the hours per month of care were collected for each of six types of informal care and formal community services (personal care, home health aide, housekeeping/home-maker, meals, transportation, financial management, arranging services/case management or social work). To collect the hours of informal care, the caregiver was queried specifically about the amount of time spent on activities that were necessary because of the elder's disability. Services purchased privately in addition to those provided by public and private agencies were considered formal services to capture more completely the use of formal care. Hours per month for each type of informal care and formal services were summed to obtain total hours per month of informal and formal care respectively. In the case of missing data for hours of care (i.e., caregiver was not interviewed), hours of care were estimated using multiple model-based imputation (Crawford et al., 1995).

Statistical Analysis

The study sample used in these analyses consisted of the 483 disabled elders with caregivers. The comparison among three ethnic groups in the elder and caregiver characteristics was performed using the Pearson χ^2 statistics for categorical variables and analysis of variance (ANOVA) for continuous variables. Both the receipt of informal care and formal services (yes/no) and the amount of help received (hours per month) were compared among three ethnic groups. A multiple logistic regression model was used for the former comparison. A multiple linear regression model was used for the latter comparison for elders who received non-zero hours of help. The hours of help received was log transformed due to the skewness of the distribution. The covariates included in the multiple regression model were those which were previously identified from the univariate analysis as well as from related work (Tennstedt et al., 1990, 1993) to be significantly associated with the amount of help received. Separate regression analyses were performed for all types of informal care combined, all types of formal service combined and individual types of informal care and formal service.

RESULTS

Sample Characteristics

The characteristics of the disabled elders and primary caregivers in this study are displayed in Table 2, with statistically significant between-group differences indicated. The disabled elders in the three groups are similar in gender and age. The Puerto Ricans differ from the African-Americans and non-Latino Whites in several ways. They are lowest in terms of social class and least likely to be married. African-Americans are also not likely to be married whereas over half of the White respondents were married. Puerto Rican elders are the most disabled. Yet they report having fewer caregivers as well as fewer potential caregivers compared to the other two groups (although the latter difference is not statistically significant).

The caregivers of these elders differ across the three groups. There are significant age differences with White caregivers being the oldest and Puerto Rican caregivers the youngest. Most African-American and Puerto Rican elders have female primary caregivers, typically offspring. White caregivers, on the other hand, include almost as many men as women, as they are more frequently the spouse of the care recipient. For similar reasons, they are also more likely to live with the care recipient. Interestingly, Puerto Rican elders, although the most disabled, are least likely to live with their caregiver. These caregivers had been providing care for a considerable period of time (6-7 yrs) with no significant between-group differences in duration of care. Finally, Puerto Rican caregivers were least likely to be employed whereas African-American caregivers were the most likely of the three groups to be employed.

Informal Care

As indicated in Table 3, disabled elders in all three groups reported receiving a variety of informal care. Help with instrumental activities of daily living (IADL) was received more frequently than help with personal activities of daily living (PADL). At the bivariate level there were ethnic differences in the four types of informal care received, specifically: personal care, housekeeping, meals and arranging services. For all types, Puerto Ricans most frequently reported receipt. Similarly, for elders receiving help, there were statistically significant ethnic differences in the total hours of care received per month. Puerto Ricans received the greatest amount of care, with African-American and White elders receiving similar amounts of care.

However, after adjusting for other factors at the multivariate level, ethnicity was no longer correlated with likelihood of receiving various types of care with the exception of receipt of help with arranging services by older Puerto Ricans. Rather, the data in Table 4 indicate that extent of disability, or need

TABLE 2. Sample Characteristics: Elders and Caregivers

	African-American		Puerto Rican		White	
	%	Mean (S.D.)	%	Mean (S.D.)	%	Mean (S.D.)
ELDER	(n = 156)		(n = 214)		(n = 113)	
Gender: Female	66.7		62.6		62.8	
Age (Range: 60-105)		71.5 (8.1)		70.7 (8.1)		72.5 (8.3)
SES (Range: 0-100)***		41.6 (20.1)		27.4 (19.3)		54.1 (22.1)
Disability (Range: 1-13)***		6.1 (3.4)		6.8 (3.2)		5.2 (3.5)
Marital Status: Married***	36.5		31.8		54.0	
Number of Caregivers*						
1	46.8		53.7		47.8	
2	25.0		32.2		29.2	
3+	28.2		14.0		23.0	
Number of Potential Caregivers						
0	31.7		37.0		29.4	
1	22.0		25.5		21.2	
2+	46.3		37.6		49.4	
CAREGIVER	(n = 131)		(n = 194)		(n = 84)	
Gender: Female***	72.5		79.9		54.8	
Age (Range: 15-89)***		50.6 (16.5)		47.6 (14.1)		60.6 (13.7)
Marital Status: Married	45.0		46.9		72.6	
Employed***	51.5		25.3		39.8	
Relationship to Elder***						
Spouse	26.2		25.1		46.0	
Offspring	47.6		55.4		36.9	
Other Relative	19.5		15.2		9.9	
Non-Relative	6.7		4.3		7.2	
Co-residence with Elder*	58.8		50.5		67.9	
Duration of Caregiving		6.8 (7.3)		7.1 (7.6)		5.8 (8.1)

*** $p < .001$ ** $p < .01$ * $p < .05$
Note: Asterisks refer to statistically significant differences across the three groups.

TABLE 3. Receipt of Informal Care and Formal Services by Ethnic Group: Percent Receiving and Mean Hours

	African-American		Puerto Rican		White	
	%	Hrs	%	Hrs	%	Hrs
INFORMAL						
Personal Care**(a)	47.2	3.4	61.1	5.6	41.6	8.6
Housekeeping***	89.4	16.1	96.4	17.0	84.6	12.6
Meals**	60.4	12.7	67.4	16.6	50.0	12.5
Transportation	64.9	5.9	65.2	3.6	58.6	6.2
Arranging Services***	28.2	1.8	47.0	1.4	20.7	1.2
Financial Management	53.5	1.1	58.1	1.0	50.5	1.6
MEAN HOURS/MONTH(b)*		30.5		41.1		29.1
FORMAL						
Home Health Aide	17.2		15.7		15.9	
Housekeeping	15.3		15.8		14.5	
Meals	10.1		6.4		8.3	
Transportation**	15.9		6.0		4.8	
Case Management/Social Work*	16.9		8.3		5.3	
Financial Management	–		–		0.9	
Any of these Services	34.5		30.5		29.2	
MEAN HOURS/MONTH(b)		11.3		14.3		12.2

***p < .001   **p < .01   *p < .05
(a)Significant differences in percent receiving type of care
(b)Geometric Mean of non-zero hours

for care, as well as the source of care (i.e., gender, relationship, and sometimes coresidence of the caregiver) were related to the likelihood of receiving specific types of care. That is, greater disability and having a female caregiver increased the chances of receiving most types of help. The relationship of caregiver to care recipient appears related to likelihood of care through the effect of coresidence status. That is, coresiding offspring were less likely than spouses to provide help with personal care but more likely to help with housekeeping, meal preparation, transportation and financial management. When compared to noncoresiding offspring, they were five times as likely to help with meal preparation.

Turning to factors associated with hours of care (Table 5), generally ethnicity was not related to the amount of informal care received, either total amount or amount of each type of care when controlling for other factors. The one exception was that African-American caregivers provided less personal care than did White caregivers. In contrast to its association with likelihood of receiving care, disability or the need for care was related only to the total amount of care and the hours of personal care, i.e., greater need was

TABLE 4. Factors Associated with Receipt of Informal Care: Odds Ratios (95% Confidence Intervals)

Variable	Personal Care	Housekeeping	Meals	Transportation	Arranging Services	Financial Mgt.
Extent of Disability	1.37 (1.27, 1.48)	1.44 (1.21, 1.70)	1.23 (1.14, 1.32)		1.15 (1.08, 1.23)	1.16 (1.09, 1.23)
Ethnicity [a]						
Puerto Rican						
African-American					2.78 (1.30, 5.95)	
Caregiver Gender: Female	2.21 (1.24, 3.94)				2.20 (1.27, 3.82)	
Relationship (for coresiding CG) [b]						
Offspring	0.48 (0.24, 0.94)	11.86 (2.44, 57.55)	3.28 (1.59, 6.78)	2.96 (1.58, 5.53)		2.77 (1.52, 5.03)
Coresidence (by CG relationship) [c]						
Offspring			5.09 (2.41, 10.80)			
Other/Non-Relative		0.06 (0.006, 0.69)				

(a) Reference group: White
(b) Reference group: Spouse coresiding caregivers
(c) Reference group: Non-coresiding caregivers in each relationship subgroup

TABLE 5. Factors Associated with Log Hours of Informal Care, Total and by Type of Care[a]: Regression Coefficients (Std Errors)

	Total Hrs	Personal Care	Housekeeping	Meals	Transportation
Extent of Disability	0.10 (0.02)***	0.18 (0.03)***			
Ethnicity [b]					
Puerto Rican					
African-American		−0.97 (0.33)**			
Elder SES					
Caregiver Gender: Female	0.37 (0.16)*	0.66 (0.27)*	0.33 (0.14)*	1.14 (0.18)***	
Relationship (for coresiding CG) [c]					
Offspring	0.57 (0.18)**				
Coresidence (by CG relationship) [d]					
Offspring	0.78 (0.18)***		0.76 (0.19)***	0.82 (0.21)***	
Other/Non-Relative			0.80 (0.29)**		

*** p < .001   ** p < .01   * p < .05
[a] Financial management and arranging services excluded due to minimal hours of care
[b] Reference Group: White
[c] Reference Group: Spouse coresiding caregivers
[d] Reference Group: Non-coresiding caregivers in each relationship subgroup

associated with more care. Instead, the data indicate that the amount of informal care received was associated more consistently with the source of care. In general, female caregivers provided greater amounts of help, and less help was received from noncoresiding caregivers, regardless of ethnicity. Further, coresiding offspring provided more total hours of care then did spouses.

Formal Services

As indicated in Table 3, formal services were used much less than informal care by all three ethnic groups. The only between-group differences were for transportation and case management or social work, where more African-Americans used these services than did Puerto Rican or non-Latino White disabled elders. When services were used, relatively few hours were used, with no statistically significant between-group differences in total hours/ month. Factors associated with any use of formal services and the hours/ month of service, if used, are displayed in Table 6. Consistent with bivariate results, ethnicity was not related to service use. Rather, it was the level of

TABLE 6. Factors Associated with Use and Amount of Formal Service

	Any Service Use Odds Ratio (95% C.I.)	Total Log Hours/Month Coefficient (Std Error)
Extent of Disability	1.36 (1.26, 1.47)	0.22 (0.05)***
Coresidence (by CG relationship) [a] Offspring	0.54 (0.27, 1.07)	

***p < .001
[a]Reference group: Non-coresiding offspring

disability that was associated with both likelihood of use and hours of use. That is, having greater disability was correlated with increased odds of using services as well as using greater amounts of service. Having a coresiding offspring caregiver reduced the odds of using formal services (although the significance level was .08).

DISCUSSION

This cross-sectional comparison of Puerto Rican, African-American, and non-Latino White persons provides a snapshot of elders, part of which is consistent with previous reports and part of which is startlingly different. The sociodemographic and disability characteristics of elders in this sample are similar to what has been reported in both national and area studies. The differences occur in relation to what has been reported previously or commonly assumed about the caregiving arrangements in these three groups.

As expected, there was greater disability among the minority elders, with the Puerto Ricans being both more likely to report any disabilities and reporting greater disability than either African-American or White elders. A related comparison of actual performance (i.e., physical capacity) to self-reported disability indicated that the ethnic differences in disability were attributed largely to differences in the elder's functional limitations or physical capacity (Jette et al., 1995). That is, these ethnic differences are real and not related to cultural influences on behavior or performance of daily living activities.

What was not expected, however, was the overall lack of relationship between ethnicity and both patterns of care and amounts of care when controlling for other factors. That is, when controlling for level of disability and characteristics of the caregiving situation, the minority elders generally received similar types and amounts of both informal care and formal services as did White elders. Rather than to ethnicity, the patterns of care, including both informal and formal, across all three groups were related to the extent of disability and the characteristics of the primary caregiver. These findings regarding the minority elders are consistent with what has been reported for non-Latino Whites (Tennstedt et al., 1990,1993). However, one should not similarly assume that the stability and resilience of the informal care system will be the same for minorities as for Whites.

Data regarding the Puerto Ricans in this study merit particular attention in this regard. While the patterns of care are generally similar to that of non-Latino Whites, there are important differences for Puerto Ricans in who provides this care. Contrary to what might be expected, older Puerto Ricans reported fewer people providing them care. Given that the amount of care they received was similar to White elders who had more caregivers, this means that Puerto Rican caregivers were providing more help to a needier group of care recipients than their non-Latino counterparts. Another point to consider is that these older Puerto Ricans were less likely than either White or African-American elders to live with their caregiver. Separate residences can make the provision of care more difficult since more time is involved in both travel and maintenance of two residences. Thus, we see with these highly disabled Puerto Ricans a situation in which there is great pressure on one or two people to meet their needs with little assistance from formal services or other community supports (Delgado, 1995). Given that these elders also report fewer potential caregiving resources, they certainly appear to be a population at risk for unmet need.

It is commonly assumed that Latino families have a strong commitment to family and, therefore, are highly likely to provide care for a disabled older family member regardless of what it takes to do so. However, as evidenced for non-Latino populations (Doty, 1986; Hanley et al., 1991), there is also evidence of changing family structures and social roles for Latino that, where not affecting their willingness to provide care, might influence their availability to do so.

The "social adaptation" approach, proposed by Vega (1990) for understanding attitudinal and behavioral changes in the family lives of Hispanics, places greater attention on the social situations and contexts that affect families. Among Puerto Ricans migrating to the mainland U.S. in search of jobs, there is clear evidence of socioeconomic adaptation with associated changes in family structure and roles. These structural roles may influence the ability of families to provide elder care or to continue to provide care if need for care increases. In addition to the increased employment rate of women, other social trends influencing the availability of Puerto Rican families, and particularly women, to care for their disabled elders are also evident. As described by Ortiz (1995)

. . . Puerto Rican women have experienced the most dramatic changes in marital and family status over the last 30 years. They are less likely to

> be married, more likely to head families on their own, and more likely to have children at younger ages and prior to marriage. (p. 35)

In sum, as Puerto Rican families continue to adapt to the changing socioeconomic context of life in the mainland U.S., we cannot assume that their familism will override social demands (challenges) from external sources. That is, as identified by Bastida in 1988, we cannot assume that Puerto Rican families will be available and able to provide care for older, disabled members.

The increasing ethnic diversity as well as overall size of the U.S. elderly population make it imperative that we develop accurate estimates of demand for services for long-term care policy development. Empirical evidence indicates that both disability and provision of informal care must be considered when estimating demand (Tennstedt et al., 1993). The data from this study call into question commonly held assumptions about the role of families in providing care and its effect on use of long-term care services. It appears that structural factors may override cultural (behavioral) factors in influencing how informal care is provided and formal services are used, particularly in the minority groups. Importantly, the data raise serious questions about the future availability of informal care for the highly disabled (predominantly Puerto Rican) elders.

Social workers are in a unique position to assist Puerto Rican and other Latino elders and their informal caregivers. The findings from this study indicate a special need for social service organizations to reach out to Puerto Rican elders in need of services or to modify their services to be more responsive and receptive to this population. The underutilization of services observed in this study is not likely unique to this city, and might reflect either lack of knowledge about these services or a reluctance to use stemming from cultural factors. Service providers can work with local Latino community organizations to identify barriers to service use and ways to be responsive to meeting the needs of older Latinos. These organizations might provide space for social service providers (outstationing) which can facilitate access to elders via their geographical location, cultural understanding, and established trust and credibility in the community. Outreach to older Latinos in need of assistance can also be facilitated through other informal organizations such as grocery and retail stores (bodegas), social clubs, and houses of worship (Delgado, 1995, 1996a, 1996b, 1998). These community settings offer opportunities to identify older Latinos who are disabled and need services, and as a result, might be willing to facilitate outreach and services delivery if asked to do so. Finally, the informal caregivers of disabled elders are also in need of support and assistance. As revealed in this study, these caregivers are helping elders with high levels of disability while juggling other responsibilities and demands on their time. It is clear that the vast majority of families want to help disabled older relatives. This commitment is particularly strong in Latino families. Attention to their needs, as well as those of older Latinos, would undoubtedly be beneficial.

REFERENCES

Bastida, E. (1988). Reexamining assumptions about extended familism: Older Puerto Ricans in a comparative perspective. In Marta Sotomayer and Herman Curiel (Eds.) *Hispanic Elderly: A Cultural Signature*. Edinburg, TX: Pan American University Press.

Becerra, R., Shaw, D. (1988). *The Hispanic elderly: A research reference guide*. New York: University Press of America.

Burr, J. (1990). Race/sex comparisons of elderly living arrangements. *Research in Aging* 12(4):507-530.

Cantor, M.A. (1975). Life space and the social support system of the inner city elderly of New York. *The Gerontologist* 15:23-27.

Cantor, M.A. (1979). The informal support system of New York's inner city elderly: Is ethnicity a factor? In Gelfand, D., Kutzik, A. (Eds.). *Ethnicity and Aging: Theory, Research and Policy*. New York: Springer.

Chatters, L.M., Taylor, R.J., Jackson, J.S. (1986). Aged blacks' choice for an informal helper network. *Journal of Gerontology* 41:94-100.

Chatters L.M., Taylor, R.J., Jackson, J.S. (1985). Size and composition of the informal helper networks of elderly blacks. *Journal of Gerontology* 40:605-614.

Chesney, A.P., Chavira, J.A., Hall, R.P., Gary, H.E. (1982). Barriers to medical care of Mexican Americans: The role of social class, acculturation, and social isolation. *Medical Care* 20:883-891.

Cox, C., Monk, A. (1990). Minority Caregivers of Dementia Victims: A Comparison of Black and Hispanic Families. *Journal of Applied Gerontology* 9(3)340-354.

Crawford, S., Tennstedt, S., McKinlay, J. (1995). A comparison of analytic methods for non-random missingness of outcome data. *Journal of Clinical Epidemiology*. 48(12):209-219.

Day, J.C. (1992). U.S. Bureau of the Census. *Population Projections of the United States, by Age, Sex, Race, and Hispanic Origin*: 1992 to 2050, Current Population Reports, P25-1092. U.S. Government Printing Office, Washington, DC (middle series projections).

Delgado, M., Humm-Delgado, D. (1982). National support systems: Source of strength in Hispanic communities. *Social Work* 83-89.

Delgado, M. (1995). Puerto Rican elders and natural support systems: Implications for human services. *Journal of Gerontological Social Work* 24(1/2): 115-130.

Delgado, M. (1996a). Puerto Rican elders and botanical shops: A community resource or liability? *Social Work in Health Care*. 23,67-81.

Delgado, M. (1996b). Religion as a caregiving system for Puerto Rican elders with functional disabilities. *Journal of Gerontological Social Work*, 26,129-144.

Delgado, M. (1998). Puerto Rican elders and merchant establishments: Natural caregiving systems or simply business? *Journal of Health and Social Policy*, 30, 39-51.

Deyo, R.A., Diehl, A.K., Hazuda, H., Stern, M.P. (1985). A simple language-based acculturation scale for Mexican Americans: Validation and application to health care research. *American Journal of Public Health* 75:51-55.

Doty, P. (1986). Family care of the elderly: The role of public policy. *Milbank Quarterly* 64(1):34-75.

Eribes, R., Bradley Rawls, M. (1978). The underutilization of nursing home facilities by Mexican American elderly in the south-west. *The Gerontologist* 18:363-37.

Estrada, A., Trevino, F., Ray, L. (1990). Health care utilization barriers among Mexican Americans: Evidence from HHANES 1982-84. *AJPH* 80:27-31.

Ford, A., Haug, M., Jones, P., Roy, A., Folmar, S. (1990). Race-related differences among elderly urban residents: A cohort study, 1975-1984. *Journal of Gerontology: Social Sciences* 45(4):S163-171.

Greene, V.L., Monahan, D.J. (1984). Comparative utilization of community-based long-term care services by Hispanic and Anglo elderly in a case management system. *Journal of Gerontology* 39(6):730-735.

Hanley, R.J., Wierner, J.M., Harris, K.M. (1991) Will paid home care erode informal support? *Journal Health Policy Political Law.* 16:507-521.

Hatch, L. (1991). Informed support patterns of older African-American and white women. *Research on Aging* 13(2): 144-170.

Havlik, R.J., Liu, B.M., Kovar, M.G., Suzman, R., Feldman, J.J., Harris, T., Van Nostrand, J. (1987). Health statistics on older persons: United States, 1986. *NCHS Advance Data*, No. 125. DHHS Publication No. (PHS) 87-1409. Hyattsville, MD.

Hays, W., Mendel, C. (1973). Extended kinship relations in black and white families. *Journal of Marriage and the Family* Feb:51-57.

Hing, E. (1987). Use of nursing homes by the elderly: preliminary data from the 1985 National Nursing Home Survey. *NCHS Advance Data*. No. 135. DHHS Publication No. (PHS) 87-1250. Hyattsville, MD.

Horowitz, A. (1985). Family caregiving to the frail elderly. In Lawton, N.P., Maddox, G. (Eds.), *Annual Review of Geriatrics and Gerontology*. New York: Springer.

Jackson, J.J. (1980). *Minorities and Aging*. Belmont, CA: Wadsworth.

Jackson, J.J. (1985) Race, national origin, ethnicity, and aging. In Binstock, R.H., Shanas, E. (Eds.), *Handbook of Aging and the Social Sciences*. New York: Van Nostrand Reinhold, 264-291.

Jette, A., Crawford, S., Tennstedt, S. (1996). Toward understanding ethnic differences in late-life disability. *Research on Aging* 18(3): 292-309.

Johnson, C., Barer, B. (1990). Families and networks among older inner-city blacks. *The Gerontologist* 30(6):726-733.

Kart, C. (1991). Variation in long-term care service use by aged blacks. *Journal of Aging and Health* 3(4):511-526.

Kemper, P. (1992). The use of formal and informal care by the disabled elderly. *Health Services Research* 27:421-451.

Lacayo, C.G. (1980). *A National Study to Assess the Service Needs of the Hispanic Elderly–Final Report*. Los Angeles, CA: Asociacion National Por Personas Mayores.

Lawton, M.P., Rajagopal, D., Brody, E., Kleban, M.H. (1992). The dynamics of caregiving for a demented elder among black and white families. *Journal of Gerontology: Social Sciences* 47(4):S156-S164.

Lindholm, M.G., Lopez, R. (1980). *Fundamentals of proposal writing: A guide for minority researchers.* National Institute of Mental Health, Center for Minority Group Mental Health Programs, Rockville, MD.

Littman, M. (1991). U.S. Bureau of the Census. *Poverty in the United States*: 1990; Current Population Reports, Series P-60, No. 175. U.S. Government Printing Office, Washington, DC, Tables 2 and 3.

Lopez-Aqueres, W., Kemp, B., Staples, F., Brummel-Smith, K. (1984). Use of health care services by older Hispanics. *Journal of American Geriatric Society* 32:435-440.

Maldonado, D., Jr. (1985). The Hispanic elderly: A socio-historical framework for public policy. *Journal of Applied Gerontology* 4, 6-17.

Manton, K.G., Poss, S.S., Wing, S. (1979). The black/white mortality crossover: Investigation from the perspective of the components of aging. *The Gerontologist* 19:291-300.

Markides, K.S., Levin, J.S., Ray, L.A. (1985). Determinants of physician utilization among Mexican Americans: A three-generation study. *Medical Care* 23:236-246.

McCullagh, P., Nelder, J.A. (1989). *General Linear Models*, 2nd Edition. Chapman and Hall. Miller, B., Campbell, R.T., Davis, L., Furner, S., Giachello, A., Prohaska, T., Kaufman, J.E., Li, M., Perez, C. (1995). Minority use of community long-term care services: A comparative analysis. *Journal of Gerontology: Social Sciences*. In press.

Miller, B.H., McFall, S. (1991). The effect of caregiver's burden on change in frail elder persons' use of formal helpers. *Journal of Health and Social Behavior* 32, 165-179.

Miller, B., McFall, S., Campbell, R.T. (1994). Changes in the sources of community long-term care among African-Americans and White Frail Older Persons. *Journal of Gerontology: Social Sciences* 49:514-524.

Mindel, C.H., Wright, R., Starrett, R.A. (1986). Informal and formal health and social support systems of black and white elderly: A comparative cost approach. *The Gerontologist* 26:279-85.

Mitchell, J., Register, J.C. (1984). An exploration of family interaction with the elderly by race, socioeconomic status, and residence. *The Gerontologist* 24:48-54.

Morrison, B.J. (1983). Sociocultural dimensions: Nursing homes and the minority aged. In George S. Getzel and Joanna M. Mellor (Eds.), *Gerontological Social Work Practice in Long-Term Care.* New York: The Haworth Press, Inc.

Mutchler, J. (1990). Household composition among the non-married elderly. *Research in Aging* 12(4):487-506.

Nam, C., Power, M. (1983). *The socioeconomic approach to status measurement.* Houston: Cap and Gown Press.

Neighbors, H., Jackson, J. (1984). The use of informal and formal help: Four patterns of illness behavior in the black community. *American Journal of Community Psychology* 12:629-644.

Reuben, D.B., Siu, A.L. (1990). An objective measure of physical function of elderly outpatients: The physical performance test. *Journal of the American Geriatrics Society.* 38:1105-1112.

Sanchez-Ayendez, M. (1988). Elderly Puerto Ricans in the United States. In Applewhite, S. (Ed.), *Hispanic Elderly in Transition: Theory, Research, Policy and Practice.* New York: Greenwood Press.

Sanchez-Mayers, M. (1985). Hispanic cultural resources for prevention and self-help. In Maldonado, D., Applewhite, S. (Eds.), *Cross-cultural Social Work Practice in Aging: A Hispanic Perspective.* Arlington, TX: The University of Texas at Arlington.

Shanas, E. (1979). Social myth as hypothesis: The case of family relations of old people. *The Gerontologist* 19:3-9.

Short, P., & Leon, J. (1990). *Use of home and community services by persons ages 65 and older with functional difficulties.* National Medical Expenditure survey research findings 5, Agency for Health Care Policy and Research. Rockville, MD, Public Health Service.

Sokolovsky, J. (1990). Bringing culture back home: Aging, ethnicity, and family support. In Jay Sokolovsky (Ed.), *The Cultural Context of Aging.* New York: Bergin and Garvey.

Soldo, B.J., Agree, E., Wolf, D. (1989). The balance between formal and informal care. In Ory, M., Bond, N. (Eds.), *Aging and Health Care.* London: Routledge.

Soldo, B.J. (1985). In-home services for the dependent elderly: Determinants of current use and implications for future demand. *Research in Aging* 7:281-304.

Solis, J.M., Marks, G., Garcia, M., Shelton, D. (1990). Acculturation, access to care, and Hispanics' use of preventive health services. *Am J Public Health* 80(Suppl):11-19.

Sotomayor, M. (1973). A study of Chicano grandparents in an urban barrio. Unpublished doctoral dissertation, School of Social Work. Denver, CO: University of Denver.

Stone, R., Cafferata, G.L., Sangl, J. (1987). Caregivers of the frail elderly: A national Profile. *The Gerontologist* 27(5):616-626.

Taylor, R.J. (1985). The extended family as a source of support to elderly blacks. *The Gerontologist* 25:488-495.

Tennstedt, S.L., Crawford, S.L., McKinlay, J.B. (1993). Is family care on the decline? A longitudinal investigation of the substitution of formal long-term care services for informal care. *The Milbank Quarterly* 71:601-624.

Tennstedt, S., McKinlay, J. (1989). Informal care for frail older persons. In Ory, M. and Bond, K. (Eds.), *Aging and Health Care.* London: Routledge.

Tennstedt, S., Sullivan, L., McKinlay, J., D'Agostino, R. (1990). How important is functional status as a predictor of service use by older people? *Journal of Aging and Health* 2(4):439-461.

Tennstedt, S., McKinlay, J., Crawford, S. (1993). Kinship tie vs. coresidence: Predictors of patterns of care. *Journal of Gerontology: Social Sciences* 48(2):S74-S83.

Trevino, F.M., Moss, A.J. (1984). Health indicators for Hispanic, black, and white Americans. *Vital and Health Statistics Series* 1984; 10(148), DHHS Pub. No. PHS 84-1576. Washington, DC: Public Health Service, National Center for Health Statistics.

Trevino, F.M., Moss, A.J. (1983). Health insurance coverage and physician visits among Hispanic and non-Hispanic people. In *Health-United States*. DHHS Pub. No. PHS 84-1232. Washington, DC: DHHS PHS, NCHS, 45-48.

U.S. Bureau of the Census. (1991). *Data for 1990, from 1990 Census of Population.* CPHL-74, Modified Age and Race Count. Washington, DC: Government Printing Office.

U.S. Bureau of the Census. (1989). The Hispanic population in the United States: March 1988. *Current Population Reports*; Series P-20, no. 438. Washington, DC.

Van Nostrand, J.F., Furner, S.E., Suzman, R., eds. (1993). Health data on older Americans: United States, 1992. National Center for Health Statistics. Vital Health Stat 3(27).

Vega, W.A. (1990). Hispanic families in the 1980s: A decade of research. *Journal of Marriage and the Family* 52:1015-1024.

Wallace, S.P., Campbell, K., Lew-Ting, C.Y. (1994). Structural barriers to the use of formal in-home services by elderly Latinos. *Journal of Gerontology* 49:5253-5263.

Wallace, S.P., Facio, E.L. (1987). Moving beyond familism: Potential contributions of gerontological theory to studies of Chicano/Latino aging. *Journal of Aging Studies* 1:333-354.

Wallace, S.P., Storms, L.L., Ferguson, L.R. (1995). Access to paid in-home assistance among disabled elderly people: Do Latinos differ from non-Latino Whites? *American Journal of Public Health* 85(7): 970-975.

Zinn, M.B. (1995). Social science theorizing for Latino families in the age of diversity. In Zambrana, R. (Ed.), *Understanding Latino Families*. Thousand Oaks, CA: Sage.

Index

In this index, page numbers followed by "t" designate tables.

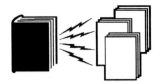

Haworth
DOCUMENT DELIVERY
SERVICE

This valuable service provides a single-article order form for any article from a Haworth journal.

- *Time Saving:* No running around from library to library to find a specific article.
- *Cost Effective:* All costs are kept down to a minimum.
- *Fast Delivery:* Choose from several options, including same-day FAX.
- *No Copyright Hassles:* You will be supplied by the original publisher.
- *Easy Payment:* Choose from several easy payment methods.

Open Accounts Welcome for . . .
- Library Interlibrary Loan Departments
- Library Network/Consortia Wishing to Provide Single-Article Services
- Indexing/Abstracting Services with Single Article Provision Services
- Document Provision Brokers and Freelance Information Service Providers

---

MAIL or *FAX* THIS ENTIRE ORDER FORM TO:

Haworth Document Delivery Service
The Haworth Press, Inc.
10 Alice Street
Binghamton, NY 13904-1580

or FAX: 1-800-895-0582
or CALL: 1-800-429-6784
9am-5pm EST

PLEASE SEND ME PHOTOCOPIES OF THE FOLLOWING SINGLE ARTICLES:

1) Journal Title: _____

   Vol/Issue/Year: _____ Starting & Ending Pages: _____

   Article Title: _____

   _____

2) Journal Title: _____

   Vol/Issue/Year: _____ Starting & Ending Pages: _____

   Article Title: _____

   _____

3) Journal Title: _____

   Vol/Issue/Year: _____ Starting & Ending Pages: _____

   Article Title: _____

   _____

4) Journal Title: _____

   Vol/Issue/Year: _____ Starting & Ending Pages: _____

   Article Title: _____

   _____

(See other side for Costs and Payment Information)

COSTS: Please figure your cost to order quality copies of an article.

1. Set-up charge per article: $8.00
   ($8.00 × number of separate articles) _____

2. Photocopying charge for each article:

   1-10 pages: $1.00 _____

   11-19 pages: $3.00 _____

   20-29 pages: $5.00 _____

   30+ pages: $2.00/10 pages _____

3. Flexicover (optional): $2.00/article _____

4. Postage & Handling: US: $1.00 for the first article/
   $.50 each additional article _____

   Federal Express: $25.00 _____

   Outside US: $2.00 for first article/
   $.50 each additional article _____

5. Same-day FAX service: $.50 per page _____

   GRAND TOTAL: _____

METHOD OF PAYMENT: (please check one)

❏ Check enclosed ❏ Please ship and bill. PO # _____
   (sorry we can ship and bill to bookstores only! All others must pre-pay)

❏ Charge to my credit card: ❏ Visa; ❏ MasterCard; ❏ Discover;
   ❏ American Express;

Account Number:_____ Expiration date:_____

Signature: *X* _____

Name: _____ Institution: _____

Address: _____

_____

City: _____ State:_____ Zip:_____

Phone Number: _____ FAX Number: _____

MAIL or *FAX* THIS ENTIRE ORDER FORM TO:

Haworth Document Delivery Service	**or FAX:** 1-800-895-0582
The Haworth Press, Inc.	**or CALL:** 1-800-429-6784
10 Alice Street	(9am-5pm EST)
Binghamton, NY 13904-1580	